Practical Bovine Immunology

John Ellis • Victor Cortese

Practical Bovine Immunology

Hands-on Applications and Immunological Concepts

Springer

John Ellis
Department of Veterinary Microbiology,
Western College of Veterinary Medicine
University of Saskatchewan
Saskatoon, SK, Canada

Victor Cortese
Cortese Veterinary Consulting
Murrells Inlet, SC, USA

ISBN 978-3-032-15030-1 ISBN 978-3-032-15031-8 (eBook)
https://doi.org/10.1007/978-3-032-15031-8

Book cover image by Evanna Lai.

Editorial Contact: Annette Klaus
This Springer imprint is published by the registered company Springer Nature Switzerland AG
The registered company address is: Gewerbestrasse 11, 6330 Cham, Switzerland

We dedicate this book to our grandchildren Edith May, Ellie, Lena, and Liam, who keep us young and are our hope for the future.

Preface

Immunology is a subject that many, if not most veterinary students, bovine specialists, and practicing veterinarians, find difficult to understand, and to some it can be tedious, filled with obscure terms and jargon. Due to its fundamental basis in veterinary medicine, immunology is still mostly taught as a standalone course or incorporated into systems courses in the first years of the veterinary curriculum. Many students consider the subject to be a necessary requisite to complete their degree but cannot wait to put the course behind them on their way to more glamorous classes in clinical sciences. There are good reasons for these sentiments. Immunology is a detail-dense subject; details most find seemingly clinically irrelevant. This "basic science" is awash with technical jargon and acronyms, making its relevance unclear to the typical veterinary student. Nevertheless, upon any reflection, it is apparent that for health professionals of all stripes to effectively deal with and control epidemics from SARS-CoV-2 to avian influenza in cattle, a working knowledge of immunology is required. The field of immunology continues to be an area of intense research. This not only includes expanding our knowledge of this complex system and how it interacts with other systems in the body, but also how it can be used to prevent and treat bodily disorders. Originally focusing on infectious diseases, this has expanded to prevention and treatment of cancer, autoimmune diseases, arthritis, and other noninfectious syndromes. Thus, those working with cattle find themselves dealing daily with the application of immunologic concepts. They are key to understanding the application of vaccines and other therapeutics to their patients, and in discussing evidence-based studies with their clients.

Currently, there are several very good and detailed textbooks on general and veterinary immunology. It is not the objective of this book to replace or duplicate those, as they continue to be good reference sources. Rather this book is structured with the veterinary student in their clinical years and practicing bovine veterinarian in mind; a busy person who has some background knowledge of immunology, but who has forgotten many of the details, and wants a practical palatable refresher of basic and new concepts as they apply to the practice of bovine medicine.

This book is divided into two parts. The first part is a review of basic immunology as it applies to all mammals, but with examples of important species differences as they relate to cattle. It is concept-focused, with enough detail to provide a basic working understanding of the subject. The second part of the book is systems-focused, emphasizing topics that are more specific to bovine immunology. It is a more detailed review of immunological issues and recent advances that are particularly relevant to a bovine practitioner, ones that other textbooks address in a more limited manner.

Each chapter includes a typical case study that focuses on the key concepts covered in the chapter, followed by a few questions that apply those concepts to practical situations. Answers to the questions are provided in the Appendix. We hope that this more user-friendly approach will be a useful supplement to already existing immunology textbooks and fills a void for those working with cattle.

Saskatoon, SK, Canada — John Ellis
Murrells Inlet, SC, USA — Victor Cortese

Acknowledgments

This book would not be possible without our families. Thank you for your love and support.

To the many colleagues, co-researchers, and cattle owners, you have our thanks and respect for all you do.

To Dr. Michael Lairmore, who endured reading these chapters, blending our two styles of writing, while adding many useful comments on content and approach, you have our deep gratitude!

Finally, to the Springer publishing family who patiently waited for our completion of this book and guided us through this process. We did it together, thank you.

Competing Interests The authors have no competing interests to declare that are relevant to the content of this manuscript.

Contents

About the Authors

John Ellis DVM, PhD, Dipl ACVP, Dipl ACVM (immunology, virology) graduated from the University of Illinois with his doctorate in veterinary medicine in 1979. After a year in mixed practice, he completed a pathology residency and Ph.D. at Colorado State University in 1984. He was then a postdoctoral fellow at the International Laboratory for Research on Animal Disease in Nairobi, Kenya, where he worked on bovine cellular immunology. After that he was a diagnostic pathologist in the Department of Veterinary Science at the University of Wyoming. Since 1992, he has been a Professor in the Department of Veterinary Microbiology at the Western College of Veterinary Medicine, University of Saskatchewan, where he teaches virology and immunology. He is extensively published, having written or co-authored more than 200 peer-reviewed articles, and was the number 2 most cited author in veterinary literature from 1995 to 2005. He has also authored textbook chapters, and numerous papers and lectures published in conference proceedings. He has given over 300 invited lectures in various scientific professional forums. He has conducted primary research on a variety of infectious diseases ranging from lentiviral infections in sheep to cirovirus infections in pigs. One of his primary research interests has been the development and efficacy testing of intranasal and parenteral vaccines for respiratory infections, including bovine respiratory syncytial virus in calves. He is a Diplomate of the American College of Veterinary Pathologists and the American College of Veterinary Microbiology (ACVM; Immunology, Virology). He was recognized as the Distinguished Veterinary Microbiologist for 2024 by the ACVM.

Victor Cortese D.V.M., Ph.D., Dipl. ABVP (dairy) graduated from Michigan State University with his doctorate in veterinary medicine in 1980. He then entered a mixed animal/dairy practice in Wisconsin. He then moved to the veterinary pharmaceutical industry where he held various positions and had worldwide responsibility supporting cattle and veterinary vaccines, and immunology. He has also held non-tenured adjunct professor positions with the University of Wisconsin-Madison, College of Veterinary Medicine, and University of Kentucky. He currently is the owner of Cortese Veterinary Consulting LLC where he works with veterinarians and cattle producers around the world. He has many publications on viral infections, immunology, neonatal immunology, vaccination programs, bacterial infections, and young dairy calf management; several textbook chapters; and guest lectures at many veterinary, producer, and university meetings. He received his diplomat status to American Board of Veterinary Practitioners (Dairy Practice Specialty) in 1995. In September 1997, at the American Association of Bovine Practitioners Conference in Montreal, he received the AABP's Award for Excellence. In 1999, he successfully completed his Ph.D. in Microbiology from the Western College of Veterinary Medicine, University of Saskatchewan. In 2013, Bovine Veterinarian Magazine selected Dr. Cortese as 1 of the 20 most influential cattle veterinarians in the United States.

Abbreviations

ACE	Antigen capture ELISAs
AGID	Agar gel immunodiffusion test
AI	Artificial insemination
APC	Antigen-presenting cell
APP	Acute phase proteins
B	Bursal (bursa)
BALT	Bronchus-associated lymphoid tissue
BCoV	Bovine coronavirus
BCR	B cell receptor
bG-CSF	Bovine granulocyte colony stimulating factor
BHV-1	Bovine herpesvirus -1
BLV	Bovine leukemia virus
BPI3	Bovine parainfluenza 3
BRDC	Bovine respiratory disease complex
BRSV	Bovine respiratory syncytial virus
BVDV	Bovine viral diarrhea virus
C	Complement
CD	Cluster of differentiation
CFT	Complement fixation tests
CLRs	C-type lectin receptors
CMI	Cell-mediated immunity
CpG	Cytidine-guanosine-dinucleotides
CT	Cycle time
CTL	Cytotoxic T cells
DAMPs	Damage-associated molecular patterns
DC	Dendritic cells
DTH	Delayed type hypersensitivity
E. coli	*Escherichia coli*
EBL	Enzootic bovine leukosis
ELISA	Enzyme-linked immunosorbent assay
ET	Embryo transfer
FRT	Female reproductive tract
GALT	Gut-associated lymphoid tissue
GI	Gastrointestinal

GM-CSF	Granulocyte-macrophage colony-stimulating factor
GMT	Geometric mean titer
IFN	Interferon
IL	Interleukin
LCA	Leucocyte common antigen
LPS	Lipopolysaccharides
Mab	Maternal antibodies
MDCs	Ovarian monocyte derived cells
MHC	Major histocompatibility complex
MID	Minimum immunizing dose
MLV	Modified live virus (viral)
mRNA	Messenger RNA
NK	Natural killer
NLRs	NOD-like receptors
OD	Optical density
OSCs	Ovarian germline stem cells
PCR	Polymerase chain reaction
PEM	Protein-energy malnutrition
PGF2α	Prostaglandin F2α
PI3	Parainfluenza 3
PPD	Purified protein derivative
PRRs	Pathogen recognition receptors
RBPT	Rose Bengal Plate Test
RESP-RT	Respiratory and reproductive
RLRs	RIG-I-like receptors
ROS	Reactive oxygen species
SN	Serum neutralization
Str	*Streptococcus*
T	Thymic (thymus)
TB	Tuberculosis
TCM	Central memory T cells
TEF	Effector memory T cells
TGFβ	Transforming growth factor beta
Th	Helper T cell
TLR	Toll-like receptors
TNF	Tumor necrosis factor
TP	Serum total protein
Tregs	Regulatory T cells
TRM	Tissue-resident memory T cells
VNT	Virus neutralization tests

Part I

The Basics

Defense of the Body: Multiple Layers of Immunity

1

Abstract

Cattle, like other vertebrates, are born into a world of microbes. Microbes, including commensals and potential pathogens that inhabit the compartments of the body, comprise what is now known collectively as the microbiome. The microbiome, along with the immune system, plays an important role in the health of all animals. To defend against pathogens, cattle and other vertebrates have multiple layers of defense that include three key components: physical barriers, innate immunity, and adaptive immunity. The lymphoid system is an integrated system composed of primary lymphoid organs such as the thymus and bone marrow. These are the sites where T and B cells develop and mature and become immunocompetent. In contrast, secondary lymphoid organs, such as lymph nodes and spleen, are where these cells encounter antigens and initiate immune responses. These immune system components function to block or react to pathogens, produce responses to bodily trauma, and preserve an animal's health in a world full of challenges.

Keywords

Innate immunity · Adaptive immunity · Microbiome · Primary lymphoid organs · Secondary lymphoid organs

Key Concepts

- The *microbiome* consists of commensals and potential pathogens.
- There are *three layers of defense* of the body: physical barriers, innate immunity, and adaptive immunity.
- *Primary lymphoid organs* are where lymphocytes develop; *secondary lymphoid organs* are where immune responses occur.

J. Ellis, V. Cortese, *Practical Bovine Immunology*,
https://doi.org/10.1007/978-3-032-15031-8_1

Why an Immune System?

Cattle, like other vertebrates, are born into a world of microbes. Many, or even most, of these microbes are commensals, and together with potential pathogens comprise what is now called the *"microbiome."* The commensals in the microbiome are generally considered a key component of normal physiological function and health. Bodily compartments develop their own unique microbiome. For example, digestion in the rumen would be impossible without the complex microbial community that resides there, allowing the breakdown of ingested food substances. Other organ systems, such as the skin and respiratory tract, have their own microbiome, which may protect invasion by pathogens or assist in the maintenance of epithelial barrier functions. The microbiome is the subject of burgeoning literature that is largely beyond the scope of this book.

The immune system can be thought of as an interconnected system of layers, each dependent upon the other. When working properly, these layers allow animals to ward off pathogenic microbes and react to bodily injury from the array of insults all animals face during their lifetime. If these layers are compromised, such as when a microbe disrupts one of these layers, the redundancy of the immune system may become critical for survival. Recognition of the anatomy and function of the immune system is critical for the practice of veterinary medicine. The response of the immune system to microbial threats is the major focus of this book. Presented in context to real-world scenarios, we put the reader in the position of the veterinary practitioner deploying basic knowledge about the inner workings of the immune system while advancing bovine health.

What Are the Three Components of the Defense System?

Mammals, such as cattle, have evolved a complex interactive defense system to respond to pathogenic microbes. This defense system has often been described as having *three layers: physical/physiological barriers, innate immunity,* and *adaptive immunity*. The skin, the largest organ in the mammalian body, is the most obvious physical barrier. Less obvious are the antimicrobial effects of normal skin components, such as lipids, and antimicrobial factors produced by the skin microbiome. Although generally thought of as being inside the body, the respiratory, gastrointestinal, and reproductive tracts are also "in the barnyard," as they are essentially exposed to the outside world at their mucosal surfaces. The microanatomy and normal physiology of these tracts provide barrier functions. The *mucociliary escalator* (cellular-directed mucus flow) in the respiratory tract and *peristalsis* (coordinated smooth muscle contractions) in the intestines are exemplary of these constitutive barrier functions. The integrity of these barriers is affected by factors, such as proper nutrition to maintain cellular integrity, or conversely by environmental insults, such as air pollution, which may damage epithelial function. These can play a vital role in the life of bovine practitioners who must assess if poor air quality and inadequate ventilation in a calf barn may be altering the consistency of mucous and otherwise decreasing the function of the mucociliary escalator and predisposing to pathogen colonization of the respiratory tract. Thus, delivery of quality care means evaluation of the physiology of our animal patients, but also their environment, which could influence their ability to respond to pathogens.

If the normal, constitutive physical barriers are breached, the next layer of protection is the oldest (evolution-wise) part of the immune response, the *innate immune response*. This is essentially an *inflammatory response* comprising phagocytic cells (e.g., neutrophils and macrophages) and soluble mediators or cytokines (e.g., interleukin 1 produced by macrophages). The innate immune response is largely non-specific, in that it is a broad protective mechanism recognizing when something foreign is present and then reacts similarly to these nonspecific signals. We will discuss in more detail in Chap. 2 more about these "*danger signals.*" The innate immune response is designed to act locally for a short period of time. Prolonged and uncontrolled innate immune responses can do more harm than good. For example, in chronic bovine viral diarrhea virus (BVDV) infection in persistently infected calves, the innate response to the virus contributes to the catabolic state that is characteristic of the wasting disease in those animals. By trying to fight off the BVDV infection, these persistently infected animals are spending tremendous energy and resources breaking down the body reserves that set them behind in weight gain and other measures of health.

If the innate immune response is unable to eliminate a pathogen, the *adaptive immune response* comes into play. This is the part of the defense system that most people associate with an "immune response." For example, vaccines are designed to activate the adaptive immune response and mimic how an animal would respond to a pathogen, but in a specific and targeted manner. There are important overlapping functions between the innate and adaptive immune responses, as some level of inflammation is necessary for the development of an adaptive immune response; inflammation acts as a bridge between the two. Compared to an innate immune response, an adaptive immune response is more specific to specific parts of specific microbes. The principal actors in adaptive immune responses are antibodies and T lymphocytes and their cytokines.

What Is the Basic Structure and Function of the Immune System?

The immune system is made up of primary and secondary lymphoid organs. *Primary lymphoid organs,* such as the thymus, are where immune cells, the lymphocytes, develop, whereas the *secondary lymphoid organs*, including lymph nodes and the spleen, are where immune responses occur. Stem cells that are destined to become lymphocytes leave the bone marrow and populate the thymus and the ileal Peyer's patches. The "T" lymphocytes develop and mature in the thymus, hence the abbreviation "T." Here, there is a selection against auto-reactive lymphocytes (cells that recognize self-antigens), reducing the chances for autoimmune disease. T cells undergo positive and negative selection in the thymus (*thymic selection*), ensuring that only those with functional and self-tolerant T-cell receptors (meaning nonreactive against self) survive. T lymphocytes leave the thymus with predetermined specificities; they selectively recognize one antigen or epitope with a predetermined affinity that does not change over their lifetime.

The "B" lymphocytes get their name from the Bursa of Fabricius, the primary lymphoid organ for B cell development in birds. In cattle and many other mammals that lack a Bursa of Fabricius, the "Bursa equivalent" is the *ileal Peyer's patches*. Here, B lymphocytes develop and mature. As with T lymphocytes, B lymphocytes leave the ileal Peyer's patches with a predetermined specificity. But, in contrast to T lymphocytes, B lymphocytes continue to "evolve" over their lifetime. This means that every time a calf is vaccinated, it potentially develops a better antibody response, one that binds the antigen more tightly and efficiently. This is one reason why booster shots are important. The primary lymphoid organs are sensitive to physiological stress and infection, which means that damage to primary lymphoid organs, especially early in life, can have lifelong effects on adaptive immune responses.

Secondary lymphoid organs include lymph nodes, tonsils, and spleen, as well as more dispersed accumulations of lymphoid cells in various organ systems such as the respiratory tract and gastrointestinal tract. Here, they are usually named according to their location, for example, "bronchus-associated lymphoid tissue" or "BALT" and "gut-associated lymphoid tissue" or "GALT." Within secondary lymphoid tissues, there is generally some anatomical segregation of B and T lymphocytes. Within the cortex or B cell areas of secondary lymphoid tissue, there are often "germinal centers." This is where B lymphocyte evolution occurs. Areas surrounding the B cell areas are populated by T lymphocytes, which can be recirculated among various secondary lymphoid organs.

Your Case

One of your clients, a purebred Angus breeder who owns a large cow-calf operation, has asked you to vaccinate a group of 30 weanling calves for respiratory viruses. This is a particularly genetically valuable group of calves, so much so that she nursed them through an acute BVDV infection when they were all approximately 1 month old. While they all recovered, they all have failed to put on weight and appear undersized compared to calves born earlier in the season. You perform physical exams on several of the calves but find no obvious cause for their appearance. The examined calves are not febrile, appear to have normal appetites, have normal stools, and have normal respiratory rates.

Questions for You

1. How would you have likely determined that the calves had acute versus persistent BVDV infections?
2. What should you discuss with the owner concerning responses to vaccination in this group of calves?

Additional Readings

1. Ellis JA, West KH, Cortese VS, et al. Lesions and distribution of viral antigen following an experimental infection of young seronegative calves with virulent bovine virus diarrhea virus type II. Can J Vet Res. 1998;62:162–9.
2. Pang F, Long Q, Wei M. Immune evasion strategies of bovine viral diarrhea virus. Front Cell Infect Microbiol. 2023;13:1282526. https://doi.org/10.3389/fcimb.2023.1282526. PMID: 37900320; PMCID: PMC10613064.
3. Ross AA, Hoffmann AR, Neufeld JD. The skin microbiome of vertebrates. Microbiome. 2019;7:79. https://doi.org/10.1186/s40168-019-0694-6.
4. Vlasova AN, Saif LJ. Bovine immunology: implications for dairy cattle. Front Immunol. 2021;12:643206. https://doi.org/10.3389/fimmu.2021.643206. PMID: 34267745; PMCID: PMC8276037.

Additional Readings

Innate Versus Adaptive Immunity

2

Abstract

The immune system senses the presence of microbial invaders by pattern recognition. This ancient and evolved system of recognizing organisms that are "non-self" was vital to the early survival of animals. The patterns recognized by the innate immune response are called pathogen-associated molecular patterns, which are biochemical motifs that are not found in vertebrates. Inflammation is the result of this pattern recognition by the innate immune system. In contrast, the patterns recognized by the adaptive immune response are known as epitopes. These are usually subunits of large foreign proteins called antigens. B and T lymphocyte responses result from this pattern recognition, and the result is a more specific and targeted response to foreign invaders or non-self-antigens. These two primary systems are often engaged in a synergistic response to infections and other bodily insults that animals encounter throughout their lives. Likewise, knowledge of the adaptive immune system sets the stage for modern vaccines and other therapeutics used in veterinary practice.

Keywords

Pathogen-associated molecular patterns (PAMPs) · Pathogen recognition receptors (PRRs) · Cytokines · Sickness behavior · Antigens · Epitopes

Key Concepts

- The immune system senses the presence of microbial invaders by *pattern recognition.*
- The *innate immune response* is triggered by recognition of *pathogen-associated molecular patterns*—conserved biochemical motifs that are not found in vertebrates. This allows the innate immune system to recognize pathogens and thus protect the host from infection by initiating inflammation.

J. Ellis, V. Cortese, *Practical Bovine Immunology*,
https://doi.org/10.1007/978-3-032-15031-8_2

- The *adaptive immune response* is triggered by recognition of *epitopes*—usually as subunits of large foreign proteins called *antigens*. The result is *B* and *T lymphocyte* responses. By evolving to be more specific combined the ability of "memory" cells that recognize previous triggers, this arm of the immune system "adapts" and targets pathogens in a focused manner.

How Does the Immune System Recognize the Microbial World?

It is all about the *recognition of patterns* that are foreign to the body. This is accomplished through a common biochemical scheme, ligand–receptor interactions—the formation of electrostatic bonds between two complementary molecules, based on shape and charge. It is the same in the immune response, except that innate and adaptive immune responses involve different ligands and receptors to trigger responses in participating cells.

What Patterns Trigger an Innate Immune Response?

The patterns or ligands that trigger innate immune responses are structurally conserved biochemical patterns or motifs that are *not* found in vertebrates like cattle, such as lipopolysaccharides (LPS) from Gram-negative bacteria, peptidoglycan from Gram-positive bacteria, bacterial flagellin, and viral RNA. These are called pathogen-associated molecular patterns *(PAMPs)* or "*danger signals*." PAMPs are recognized by many families of receptors, such as Toll-like receptors, NOD-like receptors, RIG-I-like receptors, and C-type lectin receptors. As a group, they are called pathogen recognition receptors or *PRRs* [1–4]. They are found on the outer membrane and inside cells of the innate immune system, such as macrophages and dendritic cells, but they are also present in or on many other cell types that can become players in innate immune responses. This allows many infected cells to mount some type of innate immune response to infection, simply by being able to recognize the presence of a microbe. Cells and tissues damaged by microbes or other insults, such as trauma, release normally sequestered *damage-associated molecular patterns (DAMPs)* or "*alarmins*," such as heat shock proteins, hyaluronic acid, and peptides from collagen and elastin. DAMPs use many of the same receptors used by PAMPs. They recruit and activate phagocytic cells of the innate immune system and promote adaptive immune responses. In other words, DAMPs can contribute to the innate inflammatory milieu. Many have direct antimicrobial activity as well.

Once the bond between a PAMP and a PRR is formed, intracellular signaling pathways are triggered that leads to the expression of genes for cytokines, which are the primary soluble mediators of the immune system. These are sometimes wrongly thought of a "hormones of the immune system." While hormones and cytokines are both soluble signaling molecules, they differ markedly in their sources, targets, and roles in the body. In contrast to hormones, *cytokines* are produced mainly by *immune cells* (such as macrophages, T cells, and dendritic cells) and function primarily in the *immune system.* They act *locally or regionally*, often in a *paracrine* (on closely associated cells) *or autocrine* (on the same cell that produces them) manner, to regulate inflammation, immune responses, and cell communication. While hormones maintain homeostasis across body systems, cytokines are more involved in *rapid, localized responses* to infection, injury, or immune challenges. There are two main types of cytokines produced in an innate immune response (Table 2.1): so-called *pro-inflammatory cytokines*, notable among which are *tumor necrosis factor (TNF)-α, interleukin-1 (IL-1)*, and *interleukin-6 (IL-6)*, cause inflammation, and *Type 1 interferons (α, β)* that have direct antimicrobial effects and activate a variety of cells. The *complement system* can also be involved. A variety of microbial molecules, including bacterial cell wall components, can activate the *complement cascade* via the alternate pathway without the involvement of antibodies. When this happens, one of the components, *C5a* or *anaphylatoxin*, enhances the production of proinflammatory cytokines. Altogether, the microbe-induced production of pro-inflammatory mediators has a broad range of physiological effects, including activating phagocytic cells and lymphocytes, fever induction by direct effect on the brain, effects on vascular permeability, and protein-degrading catabolic effects. Overall, an innate immune response is essentially an inflammatory response.

Innate immune responses aimed at the elimination of invading microbes evolved to be local and transient and often go unnoticed. If a microbe spreads in the body or persists, the innate immune response switches from being protective to being pathogenic. In other words, the cytokine-mediated response effectively becomes the disease. In that case, what is observed is so-called "*sickness behavior*," which generically includes fever, anorexia, sleepiness, and depression. This is associated with the production of *acute phase proteins* (APPs), such as *haptoglobin* and *serum amyloid A*, by the liver. From a practical standpoint, measurement of APP can be used as an indicator of the severity of clinical inflammatory disease. In an

Table 2.1 Key cytokines involved in the innate immune response [5, 6]

Cytokine	Cellular sources	Biological activities
IL-1β	Macrophages, dendritic cells	Promotes inflammation, fever, and activation of lymphocytes
IL-6	Macrophages, endothelial cells	Induces acute-phase response, stimulates B cell differentiation
TNF-α	Macrophages, NK cells	Promotes inflammation, apoptosis, and recruitment of immune cells
IL-12	Dendritic cells, macrophages	Stimulates IFN-γ production by NK and T cells, promotes Th1 responses
IL-15	Monocytes, macrophages	Stimulates NK cell proliferation and survival, enhances cytotoxicity
Type I interferon (IFNs) (IFN-α/β)	Plasmacytoid dendritic cells, macrophages	Antiviral responses, activation of natural killer (NK) cells, upregulation of major histocompatibility complex (MHC) class I molecules
IL-10	Macrophages, dendritic cells	Anti-inflammatory, suppresses cytokine production, limits immune response

unresolved worst-case scenario, an organ-damaging, life-threatening "*cytokine storm*," or uncontrolled release of cytokines, can result, such as can occur in a severe septic mastitis or in a systemic response to vaccination as occurred in your case [7].

Traditionally, it was thought that, in contrast to adaptive immunity, innate immunity lacked "memory." Simply put, every time a cow sees a PAMP, it is like the first time. Now, it is thought that activation of the innate immune system can result in enhanced responsiveness to subsequent encounters with the triggering PAMPs. This process has been called "*trained immunity*." Effectively, it is innate immune memory, and it probably plays a role in host defense and pathogenic chronic inflammatory processes [2].

What Patterns Trigger an Adaptive Immune Response?

The patterns or ligands that trigger an adaptive immune response are foreign macromolecules called *antigens*, and more specifically, subunits of these macromolecules called *epitopes* or *antigenic determinants*. While PAMPs are conserved structures shared by many pathogens, most antigens are unique to a specific pathogen; however, the identification of shared antigens makes good candidates for vaccination against different variants of pathogens, such as, for example, *Escherichia coli*.

Generally, foreign proteins, fundamentally, those not recognized as self, make the best antigens; the bigger, more complex, and stable the better. Examples of potent protein antigens are clostridial toxins and bacterial flagellins. Complex carbohydrates and LPS, especially if attached to proteins, are also effective antigens, as exemplified by viral envelope glycoproteins and bacterial cell wall components and endotoxins. In contrast, simple carbohydrates and lipids make poor antigens because they are generally rapidly degraded prior to stimulating an adaptive response. The most efficacious antigens comprise multiple different epitopes, which means that many different B and T lymphocytes with predetermined specificities will react to them. In general, the number of epitopes is directly related to the size of the antigen. The response to most antigens will be *polyclonal*, in other words, involving many different clones or lineages of lymphocytes. However, some epitopes are more immunogenic than others and are said to be *immunodominant*. Regardless, specific responses by B and T cells result when lymphocytes are presented with the epitope they are destined to recognize. How they recognize invaders, and what happens then is the subject of the next two chapters.

How Do Microbes Evade the Host's Immune Responses?

Viruses and bacteria have evolved sophisticated strategies to evade the host immune system, allowing them to survive and replicate within the host. One common tactic is *antigenic variation or drift*. For example, point mutations in the genes coding for envelope glycoproteins of bovine viral diarrhea virus and bovine coronavirus lead to frequent changes in the proteins on their surface, allowing them to avoid efficient recognition by antibodies produced to an older version of the same protein. Some bacteria, such as *Mycobacterium avium* and *Brucella abortus*, can hide within host cells, effectively shielding themselves from immune detection. Many viruses produce nonstructural proteins that inhibit immune responses, such as proteins that block signaling pathways in the innate immune response essential for activating immune cells. Viruses such as bovine viral diarrhea virus (BVDV) and bovine herpesvirus-1 (BHV-1) can directly attack and disable key components of the immune system, such as macrophages and helper T cells. Additionally, both viruses and bacteria may form biofilms or enter dormant states, making them less visible or less susceptible to immune attack. These evasion mechanisms pose significant challenges for treatment and vaccine development.

Your Case

A concerned client phones you. He reports that yesterday morning, he vaccinated 21, suckling, apparently healthy, Simmental calves approximately 7–30 days of age with a combination vaccine containing inactivated bovine viral diarrhea virus, parainfluenza-3 virus, bovine herpesvirus 1, bovine respiratory syncytial virus, a *Histophilus somnus* bacterin, and an adjuvant containing mycobacterial cell wall components. The injections were delivered intramuscularly in the rear limbs. He purchased the vaccine at the feed store because he was in a rush and could not book a call with you till next week. He said it took approximately 1 h to vaccinate the calves, and he did not notice anything wrong at the time of vaccination or immediately thereafter. He checked the calves after lunch, and they all appeared normal. Later in the afternoon, approximately 10 h after vaccination, he found one of the older calves (approximately 20 days of age) dead, and the remaining 20 calves were severely depressed and listless. Calves were reluctant to stand, refused to suck, and all had large, hot swellings at the site of injection. The calves appeared stiff and sore when he tried to get them to move. He managed to get rectal temperatures from several calves, and all were >40 °C. He then easily caught 15 of the 20 calves and gave them long-acting penicillin, 33,000 IU/kg body weight, and dexamethasone. Five of the calves were not as severely depressed and escaped treatment. Early this morning, he checked the calves and thought they were back to normal; they were competing at the creep feed bunk. Last night, he did some research on the internet and thinks his calves had anaphylactic reactions to the vaccine, but wants you to come out and confirm that by doing a necropsy on the calf that died. Your necropsy reveals that the diaphragmatic lobes of the lungs were heavy, wet, and reddened. The kidneys were dark red, and there was bilateral perirenal hemorrhage. There was a slight swelling in the hindquarters where he thought he had vaccinated the calf. There were no apparent gross lesions in other organ systems.

Questions for You

1. Based on the clinical history and your necropsy findings, is this owner most likely to be correct in his "internet diagnosis" of anaphylaxis? Why or why not?
2. What is the most likely immunological mechanism involved in this case?

Additional Readings

1. Li D, Wu M. Pattern recognition receptors in health and diseases. Sig Transduct Target Ther. 2021;6:291. https://doi.org/10.1038/s41392-021-00687-0.
2. Netea MG, Domínguez-Andrés J, Barreiro LB, et al. Defining trained immunity and its role in health and disease. Nat Rev Immunol. 2020;20:375–88. https://doi.org/10.1038/s41577-020-0285-6.
3. Vrentas CE, Schaut RG, Boggiatto PM, Olsen SC, Sutterwala FS, Moayeri M. Inflammasomes in livestock and wildlife: insights into the intersection of pathogens and natural host species. Vet Immunol Immunopathol. 2018;201:49–56. https://doi.org/10.1016/j.vetimm.2018.05.008. Epub 2018 May 21. PMID: 29914682; PMCID: PMC6011229.
4. Carroll SL, Pasare C, Barton GM. Control of adaptive immunity by pattern recognition receptors. Immunity. 2024;57(4):632–48. https://doi.org/10.1016/j.immuni.2024.03.014. PMID: 38599163; PMCID: PMC11037560.
5. Lesta A, Marín-García PJ, Llobat L. A comprehensive review of the bovine immune response to pathogens. Int J Mol Sci. 2025;26:8461. https://doi.org/10.3390/ijms2617846.
6. Tizard I. How immune cells communicate. In: Veterinary immunology. 10th ed. Elsevier; 2018. p. 72–81.
7. Ellis JA, Yong C. Systemic adverse reactions in young Simmental calves following administration of combination vaccine. Can Vet J. 1997;38:45–7.

B Lymphocytes, Antibodies, and Their Responses to Invaders

3

Abstract

B lymphocytes, or B cells, and antibodies are designed to recognize extracellular invaders and their byproducts, such as toxins. To accomplish this, they recognize epitopes on intact antigens, usually proteins, triggering the adaptive immune response. Isotypes are biochemically different classes of antibodies that perform unique functions in an immune response, allowing precise targeting of epitopes of microbes. Immunological memory involves memory B cells, long-lived plasma cells, and persistence of antigen, and supports the immune response for repeated infections or those invaders that persist after initial responses. This memory response depends on the replicative strategies of the invader or, in the case of vaccination, the method and composition of the vaccine.

Keywords

B cells · Antibodies · Ileal Peyer's patches · Plasma cell · Isotypes · Class switching · Germinal centers · Somatic mutation · Neutralization · Immune exclusion

Key Concepts

B lymphocytes, or *B cells,* and *antibodies* are designed to recognize *extracellular invaders* and their byproducts, which may include *toxins*.

- *B cells* recognize specific epitopes on intact antigens, usually proteins.
- *Isotypes* are unique classes of antibodies that perform specific and targeted functions in an adaptive immune response.

Immunological memory involves memory B cells, long-lived plasma cells, and persistence of antigen. This phase may vary depending on the replication strategy of the microbial invader and, in the case of vaccines, the composition of the product.

J. Ellis, V. Cortese, *Practical Bovine Immunology*,
https://doi.org/10.1007/978-3-032-15031-8_3

How Do B Lymphocytes See Invaders?

The B lymphocytes, or simply "*B cells,*" and *antibodies*, the soluble mediators of B cell response, have evolved to recognize and eliminate or neutralize extracellular invaders and the toxins and other virulence factors they often produce [1–4]. To achieve this, they recognize these invaders and their products by specifically binding individual epitopes on *whole* antigens, usually some form of protein that makes up the invader. If the epitope is detected by these specific antibodies, they can identify an intact virus or bacteria in the lumen of a bronchiole or the intestine, or a whole active toxin in the blood or body fluids. In addition, they can also recognize glycoproteins (proteins with carbohydrate forming a complex) on viruses budding from infected cells. Some of these epitopes comprise a simple linear arrangement of a few of the amino acids that make up the protein. Others, so-called *confirmational epitopes* or determinants, are formed when amino acids on different parts of a line of amino acids are brought together by the way a protein is folded, for example, the three-dimensional arrangement of a viral envelope glycoprotein. This type of epitope is often a target for neutralizing antibodies and is held together by fragile electrostatic bonds that can be disrupted by some inactivation processes used during vaccine production. This may change the confirmation of these epitopes and thus alter the binding of antibodies produced to bind to these unique structures. This can have important implications for vaccine efficacy, as likely occurred in your case study.

Regardless of the epitope, the receptors that B cells use to recognize epitopes (their ligands) are antibodies fixed to the B cell surface. Simply put, the *B cell receptor (BCR)* is an antibody. As already discussed, each B cell leaves the ileal Peyer's patches destined to recognize one epitope, which means that the receptor antibody is also specific for that same epitope. Each one of the epitope-specific B cells and their progeny is called a *clone,* or *clonotype*. In the young calf, which has not been exposed to many infectious agents, there are relatively few clonotypes, B cells with different epitope specificities. The number of diverse clones with different antigen specificities and antigen binding affinities increases over the life of the animal, as B cells mutate in response to exposure to different antigens, including those found in the microbiome.

What Happens After B Cells See Their Antigen?

The binding of antigen is the first essential step in B cell activation, but this alone is usually insufficient to result in complete activation and eventual antibody production. For complete activation, several forms of "help" or *co-stimulation* are required, including cytokines produced by T lymphocytes, direct intercellular contact between the B cell and a "helper" T cell, and binding of complement components. In addition, a signal from a pathogen-associated molecular pattern (PAMP), such as a bacterial flagellin, endotoxin or bacterial (*CpG cytidine-guanosine-dinucleotides*) DNA is usually required for prolonging and sustaining a B cell response. This can occur because B cells express one of the families of pathogen recognition receptor (PRRs), e.g., Toll-like receptors. This cooperation between innate and adaptive immunity is critical for an effective immune response. This coordination allows for efficient recognition and clearance of pathogens. Failure of one component or alterations of these two systems can result in harmful immunologic responses, including allergic reactions and autoimmune diseases. Importantly, antigen binding to the BCR is a "tunable" signal that is affected by the characteristics of the antigen and the amount of co-stimulation. Some antigens, the so-called "*T cell independent antigens*," are able to stimulate antibody production in the absence of T cell help. Examples of these include endotoxin (lipopolysaccharide) from *Escherichia coli* and flagellin from *Salmonella* spp. Although B cells produce some antibody, the primary antibody-*secreting* cell is the *plasma cell*. Plasma cells develop and differentiate from antigen-activated B cells with the help of T cells and their cytokines.

What Is the Basic Structure of Antibodies as It Relates to Their Function?

The basic shape of an antibody, or *immunoglobulin* molecule, is a "Y" (Fig. 3.1). Two identical *heavy chains* form each side of the Y, and these are held together by disulfide bonds. On the outsides of the arms of the Y are two identical *light chains*, which are connected to the heavy chains by disulfide bonds. The arms of the Y are called the *Fab* region, and at the tips are the *antigen-binding sites*, which are biochemically highly variable. This variability allows the recognition of the wide variety of epitopes found on different invaders. The base or stem of the Y, the *Fc region*, is more conserved or constant biochemically. This region interacts with other components of the immune system, triggering a variety of responses.

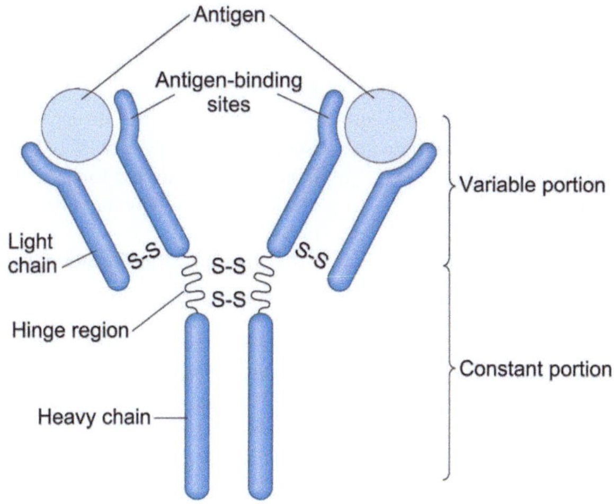

Fig. 3.1 Basic structure of an immunoglobulin. (Image Credit: periyanayagam/Shutterstock.com)

What Are Immunoglobulin "Isotypes" and How Are They Different in Function?

Antibody *isotypes* or *classes* are different forms of antibodies that play distinct roles in immune responses (Table 3.1) [1–4]. The isotype of an antibody is primarily determined by the unique biochemistry of the constant region of its heavy chain. In cattle, as is true for many other animals, there are five isotypes: *IgG, IgM, IgA, IgE, and IgD*. Isotypes or classes are sometimes further subdivided, depending on the species, into *subclasses* based on biochemical differences in their heavy chains.

IgG is the most concentrated antibody in the blood. It exists as a single Y or *monomer*, which is small enough to leak out of the vessels as a result of inflammation. The binding of IgG to an invader can clump or *agglutinate* it, and coat or *opsonize* it, both facilitating ingestion and destruction by phagocytes, such as neutrophils and macrophages. It can also *neutralize* viruses, usually by simply binding to viral surface proteins and preventing attachment and infection of host cells. Binding IgG to invaders can also trigger the complement cascade, otherwise known as *complement fixation* via the *classical pathway*. The complement system is a network of inactive proteins, principally produced in the liver, that circulate in the blood and tissues. When activated in response to infections, these proteins initiate a cascade of reactions that enhance the immune response. In cattle, there are three subclasses of IgG: IgG1, IgG2, and IgG3. In addition to being in the blood, IgG1 is predominant in some secretions, notably in colostrum and in the lower respiratory tract.

IgM is the second most concentrated antibody in the blood. When acting as a BCR attached to B cell surfaces, it is a monomer. This antibody isotype is secreted from plasma cells as a larger circular arrangement or *pentamer*, composed of five individual Ys held together by disulfide bonds and a small peptide called the *J chain*.

Table 3.1 Bovine immunoglobulin isotypes [1–3]

Isotype	Function	Key characteristics
IgM	First antibody produced in response to infection; activates complement	Pentameric structure; strong agglutination; found in blood and lymph
IgG1	Major antibody in serum; opsonization; neutralization	Dominant in response to protein antigens; Predominant isotype in colostrum, important in passive immunity
IgG2	Important in response to polysaccharide antigens; complement activation	Less efficient at opsonization than IgG1
IgA	Mucosal immunity; neutralizes pathogens at mucosal surfaces	Found in secretions (milk, saliva, tears, mucosal surfaces); dimeric form
IgE	Defense against parasites; involved in allergic reactions	Binds to mast cells and basophils; low serum concentration
IgD	Role in B cell activation (less well understood in cattle)	Primarily membrane-bound on naïve B cells

This large size means that it rarely leaves the blood even during inflammation. Because it has five functional arms, molecule for molecule, IgM is more efficient at agglutination, opsonization, neutralization of viruses, and complement fixation compared to IgG. IgM is the first isotype produced in the *primary* or first exposure to an antigen, and first, in smaller amounts, upon subsequent exposures. From a practical standpoint, this means that detection of antigen (invader)-specific IgM can be used to time exposure to an invader and detect an acute infection. This can be especially useful in vaccinated populations where antigen-specific IgG would predominate in the blood.

IgA is found primarily in secretions in the gastrointestinal, respiratory, and urogenital tracts. It is produced primarily by plasma cells under the mucosa of organs that are exposed to the animal's environment, and secreted as a dimer, two Ys held together by a J chain. It is transported through epithelial cells to lumens, where another peptide, *secretory component*, is attached to the dimer. This peptide protects the dimer from proteolytic digestion. Compared to IgG and IgM, IgA does not act as an opsonin or activate complement. Although it can neutralize viruses, it probably works primarily by agglutinating invaders and facilitating removal by the mucociliary escalator or peristalsis. This process is known as *immune exclusion*. Compared to humans or dogs, in cattle, IgA is probably less important than IgG1 as a "secretory antibody," at least in colostrum and milk.

IgE, like IgA, is primarily produced by plasma cells under mucosal surfaces. It is secreted as a monomer and mostly bound to tissue mast cells and basophils, where it acts as a *receptor*; it is present at very low concentrations in the blood. This means that IgE does not act by simply coating invaders, but rather by triggering the release of *vasoactive amines* and other soluble mediators such as serotonin, kinins, leukotrienes, and histamine, once an antigen is bound to the surface of the mast cell or basophil. Recruited *eosinophils* contribute to the inflammatory process. When IgE-mediated or *allergic* reactions occur locally, as in the case of sensitization to saliva proteins from various arthropods, such as mites, ticks, biting flies, and lice, there are the classical signs of acute inflammation, swelling, heat, redness, as well as itch. When systemic or *anaphylactic* reactions occur, the "*shock organ*" in cattle is the lung. In affected cattle, there are signs of acute respiratory distress, including tachypnea and dyspnea, accompanied by gross lesions of *atypical interstitial pneumonia*, including pulmonary edema and emphysema. As in other species, death can be averted by treatment with epinephrine and corticosteroids. Although allergies to milk, other foods, drugs, and anaphylactic reactions to vaccines are reported in cattle, IgE-mediated hypersensitivity (type 1) responses are clinically less important in cattle compared to humans or dogs, or at least they are less frequently recognized.

IgD is a monomer that is found primarily on the surface of B cells, where it is thought to be involved in B cell development. Its role in immune responses is poorly understood.

How Do B Cell Responses Change Over Time in the Individual Cow?

B cells start out having IgM and IgD as their BCR and antibody isotypes in response to an antigen. Over time, they generally change the isotype or class of the BCR and secreted antibody in a process known as *class switching*. Class switching allows the B cells and their plasma cell progeny to change the isotype of the antibody *without* changing the antigen specificity. This aids in the effectiveness of the overall response to an invader since different isotypes of antibodies have different functional processes. The process occurs in the *germinal centers* of secondary lymphoid organs and involves recombination in the genes coding for the heavy chains of the immunoglobulins. It is aided by direct contact with helper T cells and their cytokines.

Another important function that occurs in germinal centers is *somatic mutation* of B cells. This occurs by virtue of the random mutations that occur in the genes coding for the variable or *V regions* of the genes coding for the variable parts or antigen binding sites in the arms of the immunoglobulin. These mutations result in changes in the amino acids in the antigen-binding sites, either increasing or decreasing the affinity of binding. B cells that bind antigen more efficiently, that is with greater affinity, are selected for survival and clonal proliferation as a result of this *affinity maturation*. B cells that bind antigen less efficiently die by programmed cell death or *apoptosis* and are removed by macrophages. The overall outcome of this process is the generation of a diverse and efficient antibody response. Antigen-activated B cells undergo both class-switching and affinity maturation before becoming plasma cells. From a practical standpoint, every time you administer a booster shot, you provide the opportunity for somatic mutation and a potentially better antibody response to an invader.

While most somatic mutations in most cattle are beneficial, this is not always the case. An important example of pathologic somatic mutations in cancer-related genes, including TP53, KRAS, and PTEN, in cattle with *enzootic bovine leukosis*, a B cell tumor caused by the retrovirus, *bovine leukemia virus*.

How Do B Cells Remember an Invader?

Adaptive immune responses are characterized by both specificity and memory [5–9]. Primary immune responses must end; otherwise, cows and other animals would rapidly become expansive bags of antibodies. To avert this, in addition to eliminating the invader or simply removing the stimulating antigens, most antigen-activated B cells and plasma cells die by apoptosis. Germinal centers in secondary lymphoid tissues dissipate after B cell responses to an antigen have peaked.

To establish and maintain immunological memory, which is really the basis of how vaccines work, several things happen. First, in addition to activated B cells that develop into plasma cells, there is another population of B cells, sensitive to the same antigen, that persist in lymphoid tissues. They are phenotypically different, expressing different surface markers, and a protein (*Bcl-2*) that protects them from apoptosis, allowing them to become longer-lived "memory cells." Persistence of these memory cells probably best explains why there are about 10 times more plasma cells produced during a secondary exposure to antigen versus a primary exposure, as can be observed in the accelerated difference in response to a booster shot compared to a first dose of vaccine. This more rapid and quantitatively greater (antibody) response is called the *anamnestic*, literally memory, response. Second, in addition to short-lived plasma cells, which live primarily in secondary lymphoid tissues such as lymph nodes and spleen, produce antibodies shortly after exposure to an antigen, and die weeks later, there are long-lived plasma cells that live for months to years in the bone marrow. Third, persistence of antigen in lymphoid tissues can provide a long-lived source of low-level stimulation to B cells. Both latter mechanisms are often thought of as components of immunological memory.

Overall, immunological memory is still largely a black box that is incompletely understood. This is especially true when it comes to cattle and other veterinary species. Much of what we think we know has been extrapolated from studies in mice and humans. Nevertheless, one important practical implication in thinking about immunological memory is the apparent differences in the longevity of clinically effective memory to invaders with different lifestyles, or vaccines using different technologies. For example, combination vaccines for clostridial species stimulate years-long, protective antibody responses, whereas natural infections or vaccines against some acute viral infections, such as bovine herpesvirus-1, may provide only months of protection from clinical disease. Understanding the limitations of immunological memory is central to acknowledging and conveying reasonable expectations about vaccine efficacy, an important component of client relations. Remember that being "immune" is being biologically ready or primed to respond to an invader, while being clinically protected is about the prevention of clinical disease; these can be mutually exclusive and can vary with the invader [5]. This would partially explain why some vaccines appear to be better than others.

Your Case

You are consulting on a field trial evaluating a new adjuvanted subunit vaccine for bovine respiratory syncytial virus (BRSV). The vaccine is made up of a genetically-engineered whole BRSV F protein and a novel adjuvant. To ensure that all cattle in this commercial feedlot were vaccinated for BRSV, and other common respiratory viruses, you vaccinated 6-month-old calves in 5–200 head pens with the new vaccine candidate and a three-way modified-live vaccine containing bovine herpesvirus 1(BHV-1), bovine parainfluenza virus-3 (BPIV-3), and bovine viral diarrhea virus(BVDV) types 1 and 2. As a comparative "positive control," you vaccinated similar calves in five other 200-head pens with the vaccine that the feedlot has used in the past, a combination four-way modified-live vaccine containing BRSV, BHV-, BPIV-3, and BVDV types 1 and 2.

To monitor the response to vaccination, 2 weeks after vaccination, you randomly bled 10 calves from each of the pens, collected the serum, and sent it to a diagnostic lab for testing of BRSV-specific antibodies. The diagnostic lab uses a commercial enzyme-linked immunosorbent assay (ELISA) test for BRSV that has whole BRSV, purified by centrifugation in a density gradient, as the antigen.

Calves in the pens that received the new vaccine had significantly higher concentrations of BRSV-specific antibody than calves in the pens that received the four-way modified-live vaccine. You interpret these results to mean that the new vaccine is more immunogenic and may be more protective against a BRSV infection.

As luck would have it, this fall has been relatively warm and moist, good for virus transmission. Six days after a cold snap in November, the pen-riders reported increased pulls for respiratory disease. Nasal swabs were collected from all sick cattle, and quantitative polymerase chain reaction "respiratory panel" testing for BRSV, BHV-1, BPIV-3, BVDV types 1 and 2, and *Mycoplasma bovis* was done. Only BRSV was detected, and cycle threshold (CT) values in the calves that received the candidate subunit vaccine were significantly lower. At close out, the calves that had received the "control" vaccine had significantly higher average daily gains and final weights.

Questions for You

1. What do low CT values on a diagnostic PCR test report indicate? Why?
2. From the perspective of protective antibody responses alone, why do you think that the vaccine that stimulated the lower concentration of BRSV-specific antibody apparently provided better clinical protection?
3. What does the type of test that is used to quantitate virus-specific antibody tell you about the functionality of the antibody that is being measured?

Additional Readings

1. Tizard I. Antibodies. In: Veterinary immunology. 10th ed. Elsevier; 2018. p. 162–72.
2. Barroso R, Morrison WI, Morrison LJ. Molecular dissection of the antibody response: opportunities and needs for application in cattle. Front Immunol. 2020;11:1175. https://doi.org/10.3389/fimmu.2020.01175. PMID: 32595642; PMCID: PMC7304342.
3. Butler JE. Bovine immunoglobulins: an augmented review. Vet Immunol Immunopathol. 1983;4(1–2):43–152. https://doi.org/10.1016/0165-2427(83)90056-9. Erratum in: Vet Immunol Immunopathol 1985;10(1):129. PMID: 6223434.
4. Medzhitov R, Iwasaki A. Exploring new perspectives in immunology. Cell. 2024;187(9):2079–94. https://doi.org/10.1016/j.cell.2024.03.038.
5. Campos M, Godson DL. The effectiveness and limitations of immune memory: understanding protective immune responses. Int J Parasitol. 2003;33(5–6):655–61. https://doi.org/10.1016/s0020-7519(03)00066-3.
6. Ellis JA. How efficacious are vaccines against bovine respiratory syncytial virus in cattle? Vet Microbiol. 2017;206:59–68. https://doi.org/10.1016/j.vetmic.2016.11.030. Epub 2016 Dec 5. PMID: 28024854.
7. Inoue T, Kurosaki T. Memory B cells. Nat Rev Immunol. 2024;24:5–17. https://doi.org/10.1038/s41577-023-00897-3.
8. Tellier J, Nutt SL. The secret to longevity, plasma cell style. Nat Immunol. 2022;23:1507–8. https://doi.org/10.1038/s41590-022-01340-w.
9. Victoria GD, Nussenzweig C. Germinal centers. Annu Rev Immunol. 2022;40:413–42. https://doi.org/10.1146/annurev-immunol-120419-022408.

T Lymphocytes, Cytokines, and Their Responses to Invaders

4

Abstract

T lymphocytes (T cells) are important players in cell-mediated immunity. They recognize epitopes from processed antigens. These are peptides on cell surfaces presented by major histocompatibility molecules. T cell responses are designed to recognize intracellular invaders and eliminate infected cells. They also "help" in other immune responses by secreting cytokines. T cell memory involves three distinct types of memory cells: central memory, tissue resident, and effector memory cells. These components of the immune system are a major part of the adaptive immune response.

Keywords

T cells · Thymus · Major Histocompatibility Complex (MHC) · MHC restriction · Cluster of differentiation (CD) · GAMMA-delta T cells · delayed-type hypersensitivity (DTH)

Key Concepts

- *T lymphocytes (T cells)* recognize epitopes from processed antigens, peptides on cell surfaces.
- *T cell responses* are designed to recognize intracellular invaders and eliminate infected cells.
- *T cells help* in other immune responses by secreting cytokines.

T cell memory involves three distinct types of memory cells: central memory, tissue resident, and effector memory cells.

J. Ellis, V. Cortese, *Practical Bovine Immunology*,
https://doi.org/10.1007/978-3-032-15031-8_4

How Do T Lymphocytes See Invaders?

The *T lymphocytes*, or simply *"T cells,"* have evolved to recognize intracellular invaders and eliminate infected cells. Therefore, T cells are especially important in recovery from infections. They also "help" in the overall response to an invader by secreting cytokines. To achieve this, they see the invaders by recognizing individual epitopes of *processed antigens*, peptides on the surface of infected cells. They are very different than B cells in this regard. This means that they cannot directly identify an intact virus, bacteria, or parasite in the lumen of a bronchiole or the intestine, or a whole active toxin in the blood or body fluids, like B cells and antibodies can. What must happen for a T cell to sense the presence of an invader is that a cell must become infected, or an antigen-presenting cell (APC), a cell of monocyte/macrophage lineage, must ingest the invader, pieces of an invader, or its byproduct, such as a toxin. Then the antigens from an infecting or ingested microbe are degraded into peptides and are transported to the endoplasmic reticulum, where they are electrostatically bound to molecules that "present" antigens *to T cell receptors (TCRs)* on the surface of T cells. The surface of each T cell expresses many TCR molecules, all sharing the unique specificity. As with antibodies, whether soluble or fixed on the B cell surface as a B cell receptor (BCR), there is an extraordinary amount of variability in TCRs, largely because of recombination in genes coding for the TCR during T cell development in the thymus. This variability is crucial for the ability of the immune system to recognize and respond to the vast array of antigens found in microbes.

The molecules that present the processed antigens to T cells are called *Major Histocompatibility Complex (MHC) molecules.* They are so named because they were first discovered in the context of tissue compatibility and organ transplantation. They, along with the BCRs (immunoglobulin) and TCRs, belong to the immunoglobulin superfamily. Structurally and functionally, they are all somewhat similar. All the members of this family have a distinctive or modified "Y"-like shape with constant regions that bind them to cells and highly variable arm-like regions that bind antigens.

There are *two major types of MHC molecules* involved in antigen presentation, MHC Class I (MHC I) and MHC Class II (MHC II). MHC I molecules are expressed on the surface of all nucleated cells. This allows endogenous foreign antigens, such as a viral or mycobacterial protein, produced during an infection of virtually any cell to be "seen," and that infected cell can be recognized and eliminated by the immune system. In contrast, the expression of MHC II molecules is generally restricted to "professional" APCs, such as dendritic cells and monocyte/macrophages, as well as B cells, which can bind antigen via the B cell receptor (antibody fixed to the cell surface). These cells engulf exogenous antigens, such as a whole bacterium, virus, or parasite, or parts thereof, then degrade and process them, and, finally, present the resulting peptides on the cell surface attached to MHC II molecules. Dendritic cells are so-named because they are "tree-like," with long branching projections that sample the microenvironment. They are found throughout the body, including in germinal centers, and are very good at antigen presentation because they express high amounts of MHC II molecules on their cell surface. Based on these differences, MHC I molecules are said to be involved in the *endogenous pathway* of antigen presentation, whereas MHC II molecules are involved in the *exogenous pathway* of antigen presentation. Because of these requirements for presentation and recognition, T cells are said to have "MHC-restricted" responses.

How Are Different Types of T Cells Identified?

T cells, like most cells, have numerous different molecules on their cell surface, and some of these have been used to identify different types of T cells. The way this was done was to produce monoclonal antibodies against lymphocytes; antibodies that recognize one epitope. The binding of these antibodies was determined by various techniques, including immunohistochemistry and flow cytometry, imaging techniques that can identify specifically labeled cells. Once at least two monoclonal antibodies were shown to bind the same molecule on the surface of a lymphocyte, that molecule or marker was sequentially assigned *a cluster of differentiation* or "*CD*" number. In addition to being a marker for T cells and other cells, most CD molecules perform specific functions for the cells that express them. CD3 is present on all T cells as it is part of the TCR and is essential for T cell activation. It serves as a "pan T cell" marker. In cattle, there are three major subpopulations of T cells with different functions: CD4, CD8, and CD4/CD8 negative.

How Do T Cells Differ in Antigen Recognition and Functions?

Traditionally, cell-mediated immunity or "CMI" has been associated with "killer" or "cytotoxic" T cells (CTL). Virtually, all CTL in cattle express the *CD8* molecule. They can only see microbial antigens processed on infected cells if they are presented attached to MHC I molecules on the cell surface. Beyond just being a marker for CTL, the CD8 molecule acts as a necessary co-receptor that stabilizes the bond between the TCR and the MHC I-containing peptide, which the T cell specifically recognizes and responds to. Once the CTL is activated, it can kill an infected cell, for example, a parainfluenza virus-infected bronchiolar epithelial cell, by inducing apoptosis or programmed cell death, essentially "suicide". This can happen in two ways, either indirectly through the release of cytotoxic molecules, perforin and granzyme by the CTL, or directly by the CTL binding to the "cell surface death receptor," called "Fas" (CD95), on the surface of an infected "target" cell via its Fas ligand. Both require close contact between the CTL and infected target cell. This removal of cells infected with a virus or facultative intracellular bacteria, such as *Brucella abortus* or *Mycobacterium paratuberculosis*, is important in recovery from infections [1–3].

Other, often underappreciated, major players in CMI are *CD4*-positive or "helper" T cells [4]. These are the major effector cells in delayed-type hypersensitivity (DTH) reactions to *Mycobacteria* spp. and other intracellular pathogens ("spp" stands for "species plural," which indicates a group of species within a genus). They, like CD8-positive T cells, can only see processed antigen attached to MHC molecules on the cell surface, mostly on dendritic cells and mononuclear phagocytes. However, they recognize antigens presented by MHC II molecules, not MHC I. The CD4 molecule helps stabilize the electrostatic bond between the TCR and the antigen–MHC complex. CD4+ T cells "help" immune responses in a variety of ways, mostly via secreted cytokines. In humans and mice, helper T cells are mostly divided into two distinctive populations, *Th1 and Th2*, based on distinct differences in the cytokines they secrete. In contrast, in cattle, Th cells are more "flexible" in the cytokines they secrete and are usually designated as Th0, meaning that the same cell can secrete different types of cytokines that can help in a variety of ways. One important way that helper T cells "help" is in the co-stimulation of B cells. As with T cells, simply seeing an antigen is not enough for full activation of B cells. After a B cell sees and binds to its specific antigen through the cell surface receptor, the B cell receptor or "fixed" immunoglobulin, it internalizes and processes it. Fragments of the antigen, peptides, are then presented on MHC II molecules to helper (CD4+) T cells that provide the costimulatory signals by formation of a bond between CD40 on the B cell and CD40L on the T cell. This signaling leads to proliferation, differentiation, antibody class-switching, and development of plasma cells and memory B cells. Most important antigens of microbial invaders follow this paradigm and are T cell-dependent. Like T cells, B cells that do not get co-stimulated die by apoptosis or become anergic. Anergy is a state of immune unresponsiveness in which T or B cells fail to react to an antigen despite being stimulated. This is an important process as it maintains immune tolerance and prevents autoimmune responses. Specific anergy refers to a lack of reactivity to an individual antigen, while generalized anergy is the inability to react to any antigen.

The third major population of T cells in cattle (and other ungulates) is so-called *gamma-delta (γδ) T cells*, which are named based on the distinct biochemistry of their TCRs that are different from CD4 and CD8-positive T cells that have alpha/beta (αβ) TCRs. In addition, most γδ T cells, while expressing CD3, are double-negative for CD4 or CD8. Most express a unique transmembrane glycoprotein called "WC1." In marked contrast to mice and humans, γδ T cells comprise 15–60% of circulating lymphocytes and are also prominent at mucosal surfaces. They are the predominant T cells in young calves. Importantly, unlike CD4 and CD8-positive T cells, antigen presentation to γδ T cells usually occurs independently of MHC molecules, allowing them to directly recognize antigens without the need for processing. They can also recognize microbial pathogen-associated molecular patterns (PAMPs) using the WC1 molecule and can secrete various cytokines. Although the role of γδ T cells in immunity and response to vaccination is not completely understood, they are thought to serve as a bridge between innate and adaptive immunity. They can respond rapidly to infection, for example, to mycobacterial species, without prior sensitization, making them critical early in infection, especially in young calves. These T cells are also thought to perform immune regulatory functions. Other CD4-positive T cells that are less well defined in cattle compared to mice and humans are regulatory T cells (Tregs) and Th17 cells.

After T cells are presented with their specific epitope, to become fully activated, there must be a process of co-stimulation. *T cell activation* is a two-signal process. The first signal is the antigen-specific interaction between the TCR and the peptide epitope presented by an MHC-I or MHC-II molecule on the surface of an infected cell or APC. The second signal is interaction between CD28, a costimulatory molecule on the T cell, and CD80, a co-stimulatory molecule on an APC such as dendritic cells, macrophages, or B cells. This interaction enhances T cell proliferation and cytokine production. Without the second signal, a responsive T cell dies by apoptosis or becomes unreactive or tolerant (anergic). It is thought that this two-signal process of co-stimulation ensures that T cells only become fully activated in the presence of both antigen and danger signals. This maintains the specificity of CMI responses and prevents autoimmune reactions.

What Cytokines Do T Cells Secrete and What Do They Do?

As mentioned, cattle, unlike mice and humans, have T cells that are usually designated as Th0; however, the cytokines they produce are still talked about as being either "Th1-type" or "Th2-type" (Table 4.1). Generally, Th1-type cytokines help with cell-mediated immune reactions, whereas Th2-type cytokines help with antibody-mediated or humoral immune reactions. Important Th1-type cytokines are Interferon-gamma (IFN-γ), interleukin-2 (IL-2), and tumor necrosis factor (TNF)-α. Compared to type I interferons, IFN-α,β, which are produced in response to pathogen-associated molecular patterns as part of an innate immune response, the type II

Table 4.1 Cytokines produced by bovine T lymphocytes [5–7]

Cytokine	Function	Produced by
IFN-γ	Activates macrophages, enhances antigen presentation, promotes Th1 responses	CD4$^+$ Th1 cells, CD8$^+$ cytotoxic T cells, γδ T cells
IL-2	Promotes T cell proliferation and survival	Activated CD4$^+$ T cells
IL-4	Promotes B cell differentiation, class switching to IgE/IgG1, supports Th2 responses	CD4$^+$ Th2 cells
IL-10	Anti-inflammatory, suppresses antigen presentation and T cell activation	γδ T cells (major source in cattle), regulatory T cells
IL-17	Recruits neutrophils, promotes inflammation	Th17 cells, γδ T cells
TNF-α	Promotes inflammation, activates endothelial cells	CD4$^+$ and CD8$^+$ T cells
TGF-β (Transforming Growth Factor beta)	Immunosuppressive, promotes regulatory T cell development	Regulatory T cells, γδ T cells
IL-21	Supports B cell and T cell function, enhances cytotoxicity	CD4$^+$ T follicular helper cells
IL-6	Promotes inflammation, B cell differentiation	CD4$^+$ T cells (especially Th17), γδ T cells

interferon, IFN-γ, is produced primarily by T helper cells in response to specific antigens of an invader. This cytokine has direct antiviral effects by inhibiting viral protein synthesis and activates other cells, such as macrophages, which can then more effectively kill intracellular bacteria, such as *Mycobacteria* spp. or *Brucella* spp. Measurement of IFN-γ can be used as an indicator of an ongoing Th-1 type CMI response, for example, in response to viral or intracellular bacterial infections, such as in your case. As the name suggests, *interleukins*, commonly abbreviated as "*IL-*," are cytokines produced primarily by leukocytes and serve generally to communicate with other leukocytes. In mice and humans, more than 40 interleukins have been described, whereas in cattle, only about half that number have been identified. They have been named in the sequence of their discovery, but also, confusingly, often have other names, usually describing their activity. For example, the characteristic Th-1-type cytokine, IL-2, is also called T cell growth factor because its primary function is to stimulate the proliferation and differentiation of T cells, and to a lesser extent, B cells.

Important Th2-like cytokines include interleukins-4, 5, 10, and 13. IL-4 is central to B cell differentiation, promotes B cell proliferation and class-switching to IgG1 and IgE. IL-5 also supports B cell differentiation, as well as stimulating growth and activation of eosinophils. IL-10 is produced by CD4-positive regulatory T cells (Tregs); it is anti-inflammatory and suppresses Th1-type activity and macrophage activation. IL-13 has mostly been studied in mice and humans, but some evidence suggests that it is involved in allergic responses to parasites and allergens in cattle, promoting antibody class-switching to IgE and IgG1.

As their name implies, Th17 cells are characterized by their secretion of IL-17, which can also be secreted by γδ T cells. Compared to mice and humans, many details of the biology of this interleukin in cattle are lacking. However, it is thought, based on its increased concentrations in diseased cattle, and its ability to direct neutrophil migration, that IL-17 plays a role in various inflammatory processes, including the bovine respiratory disease complex, mastitis, and *Mycobacterium bovis* infections. Like many immune responses, it is probably a question of balance; a little IL-17 is protective, and a lot is pathogenic.

How Do T Cells Change Over Time in the Individual Cow?

Essentially, they do not, at least not in the way that B cells do. In marked contrast to B cells, T cells do not undergo somatic mutations in the variable genes coding for their surface receptors, TCRs, once they leave the thymus. It is thought that, generically in all mammals, this lack of somatic mutation assures fidelity in the recognition of foreign antigens and, importantly, averts or reduces the chances for the emergence of auto-reactive T cells and autoimmune diseases. However, like B cells and many other differentiated cells in the body, mutations can occur in T cells after they leave the thymus. But, in contrast to B cells, where somatic mutations generally improve the overall B cell response to invaders, mutations in T cells generally have a negative impact, as they are associated with senescence, immune dysregulation, immunodeficiencies, and cancer. All these phenomena are well documented in humans and are likely to occur in cattle as well, for example, lymphomas (solid tumors) and leukemia in mutated T cells have been reported in cattle.

How Do T Cells Remember an Invader?

As is the case with B cells, establishment of T cell memory is critical to mounting long-lived immunity and combating infectious disease. It is essential for effective vaccination. When a naïve T cell is presented with its antigen, and there are adequate co-stimulatory signals, effector T cells, killer or helper, develop. These are usually short-lived (days to weeks) and die by apoptosis. Some of these stimulated cells resist "suicide" and develop into long-lived (months to years) memory cells. As with memory B cells, generically, memory T cells have a different phenotype and behavior than effector T cells. They express different molecules on their surface membranes, notably different molecular forms (isoforms) of the leukocyte common antigen, CD45, which regulates activation. In addition to living longer, memory T cells are easier to activate and have enhanced functions. It is thought, based on studies in mice, humans, and cattle, that there are *three types of memory T cells*: central memory T cells, tissue-resident memory T cells, and effector memory T cells. Each of these has distinct expressions of surface molecules, functions, and migration patterns. Central memory cells circulate through the blood and secondary lymphoid tissue, such as lymph nodes. They do not have effector function but can respond rapidly and develop into effector cells. Tissue resident memory cells are in various tissues and can rapidly secrete cytokines in response to an invader. They do not circulate in the blood. Effector memory cells are home to sites of inflammation where they can immediately respond to an invader without having to differentiate.

Perhaps the best and most clinically relevant, readily observable example of a memory T cell response is the tuberculin skin test—a classical delayed-type hypersensitivity *(DTH)* or type IV hypersensitivity reaction. This reaction occurs 12–72 h after exposure to a recall antigen, in the case of a previously exposed cow, intradermal (tailfold) inoculation of purified protein derivative from *M. bovis*. The reaction site is composed primarily of IFNγ secreting CD4+ T cells and activated macrophages. If an intracellular infection persists, for example, in tuberculosis (TB) in humans and cattle, a DTH reaction can become a granuloma, the characteristic lesion of pulmonary TB. It is essentially a more organized, walled-off (by fibrosis) DTH reaction with prominent activated macrophages and, often, multinucleated giant cells; a chronic inflammatory response. In fact, DTH reactions as an indicator of a CMI memory response can be observed in a variety of infections ranging from BRSV to *Brucella* spp., as in your case, by similar intradermal inoculation of the relevant antigen.

Your Case

You are volunteering your services to evaluate a new vaccine to more safely and better control brucellosis in bison in Yellowstone National Park and hopefully further reduce the chances for spillover infections into cattle. You remember that there is a live attenuated vaccine, RB51, that is sometimes used by accredited veterinarians to control brucellosis. It largely replaced the older "Strain 19" vaccine, mostly because of safety concerns. The new vaccine is a subunit vaccine that is a combination of three outer membrane proteins with an oil-based adjuvant. This is quite a bit different from the current vaccine, and you are wondering if it could actually work. You are also thinking about how to best monitor the response to the vaccine in the bison, since handling them is obviously not going to be a trivial pursuit. One of the wildlife biologists you are working with remembers that skin fold tests were used to monitor TB infections in elk. She is wondering if something like that could be used to monitor responses to Brucella vaccines, and since she is a curious person, she asks you what is actually going on, from an immunological perspective, in the lump in the skin fold in *M. bovis*-exposed elk. You are thinking that even if a skin fold test could be adapted to *Brucella*, it would still require handling the bison twice after vaccination, and you are wondering if there might be another test of immunity that would require only one time through the chute after vaccination. Why not test for antibodies to *Brucella*?

Questions for You

1. You are thinking about the type of vaccine needed to be effective against *B. abortus*. Since *Brucella* spp. are bacteria, shouldn't an antibody response be sufficient? Why do we need a modified-live vaccine to begin with?
2. What specific types of immune responses would you expect to get in response to the RB-15 vaccine? Would it be the same or different with a subunit vaccine? Can an inactivated or subunit vaccine stimulate a cell-mediated or "CMI" response? Why or why not?
3. Could a skin fold test be used to monitor response to *B. abortus* vaccine? Why or why not? Answering the wildlife biologist's question, what specific types of immune responses are occurring in the lump in a positive skin fold test? Would a test for antibody be just as good?

Additional Readings

1. Heidary M, Dashtbin S, Ghanavati R, Mahdizade Ari M, Bostanghadiri N, Darbandi A, Navidifar T, Talebi M. Evaluation of brucellosis vaccines: a comprehensive review. Front Vet Sci. 2022;9:925773. https://doi.org/10.3389/fvets.2022.925773. PMID: 35923818; PMCID: PMC9339783.

2. Hogg AE, Parsons K, Taylor G, Worth A, Beverley P, Howard CJ, Villarreal-Ramos B. Characterization of age-related changes in bovine CD8+ T cells. Vet Immunol Immunopathol. 2011;140:47–54.
3. Kandel A, Li L, Hada A, Xiao Z. Differential expression of CD45RO and CD45RA in bovine T cells. Cells. 2022;11(11):1844. https://doi.org/10.3390/cells11111844.
4. Sterle H, Putz EJ, Olsen SC, Boggiatto PM. Induction of CD4 T cell memory responses following BCG vaccination of cattle. Front Vet Sci. 2024;11 https://doi.org/10.3389/fvets.2024.1491424.
5. Lesta A, Marín-García PJ, Llobat L. A comprehensive review of the bovine immune response to pathogens. Int J Mol Sci. 2025;26:8461. https://doi.org/10.3390/ijms2617846.
6. Tizard I. How immune cells communicate. In: Veterinary immunology. 10th ed. Elsevier; 2018. p. 72–81.
7. Tizard I. Helper T cells and their response to antigens. In: Veterinary immunology. 10th ed; 2018. p. 132–45.

5 Immunodiagnostics

Abstract

Immunologic testing in veterinary medicine is primarily used to diagnose exposure to microbes by measuring antibodies in serum, commonly known as serology. Numerous methodologies, including agglutination tests, neutralization tests, and enzyme-linked immunosorbent assays (ELISA), are principal tests commonly used to identify and quantitate pathogen-specific antibodies. They serve different purposes and provide unique information concerning the immune response of animals. Antigen capture ELISAs have more limited use in the diagnosis of some infections, such as bovine viral diarrhea virus (BVDV) and *Mycobacterium bovis*. Collectively, these tests form the typical panel of probes to investigate animal infections and are commonly offered together in commercial and government laboratories.

Keywords

Sensitivity · specificity · Agar gel immunodiffusion (AGID) test · Enzyme-linked immunosorbent assay (ELISA) · virus neutralization (VN) test · Capture ELISA

Key Points

- Diagnosis of infectious disease can take the form of *detecting the agent* or detecting the immunologic *response to the microbe*.
- The primary use of commercially available immunologic tests in the diagnosis of infectious disease is detecting an antibody response to the microbe by *serological testing*.
- *Agglutination* tests, *neutralization* tests, and *enzyme-linked immunosorbent assays (ELISAs)* are commonly used methodologies to measure antibody

J. Ellis, V. Cortese, *Practical Bovine Immunology*,
https://doi.org/10.1007/978-3-032-15031-8_5

responses and together indicate unique information (e.g., exposure vs. effective) of the functionality of the animal's response.
- *Antigen capture ELISAs* have more limited use in the diagnosis but are useful to identify some infections, such as BVDV and *Mycobacterium bovis*.

What Is the Difference Between Sensitivity and Specificity?

Sensitivity and specificity are the two critical measures of a diagnostic test's performance, but there is a trade-off between the two. Importantly, both are dependent on the validity of the "gold standard" that is being used to calculate them. *Sensitivity* measures a test's ability to correctly identify individuals who *have* the disease or have been exposed to a microbe. Since it is a very inclusive measure, it is also known as the *true positive rate*. Thought of differently, a highly sensitive test minimizes false negatives but increases the chances of false positives. In contrast, *specificity* measures a test's ability to correctly identify individuals who *do not* have the disease or who are less likely to have been exposed. It is also called the *true negative rate*. A highly specific test minimizes false positives but increases the chances of false negatives. An ideal test has 100% sensitivity and specificity, but this is rarely the case for diagnostic tests do to a number of factors, including antigen preparations, operator proficiency, and so on.

From a practical standpoint, for example, in eradicating BVDV from a herd, choosing between sensitive and specific tests depends on the stage of the program, but, generally, a sensitive test is more useful initially, whereas a specific test is more useful in the final stages of the program. That is because early on, the priority is to identify and remove as many infected individuals as possible, even at the risk of having some false positives. Use of a sensitive test ensures that few infected individuals or reservoirs, in this case, persistently infected (PI) calves, may be missed. After the initial stages, as infection or disease becomes rare, the priority shifts to avoiding unnecessary culling. True cases need to be confirmed, and a specific test that minimizes false positives and targets truly infected animals is, therefore, the best choice.

What Are the Two Primary Approaches to Diagnosing Infectious Diseases?

The primary use of immunological tests in bovine medicine is in the diagnosis of infectious diseases. Immunologic tests are commonly used to diagnose immune-mediated disorders in small animals and for horses. Because of practical economic relevance, immunologic tests are typically restricted to the identification of infectious agents; exceptions may occur for valuable breeding stock. Traditionally, two primary approaches have been used to diagnose infectious diseases: detection of the agent and detection of a response to the agent, either antibodies or cytokines

Table 5.1 Comparison of antibody detection tests [1–3]

Test type	Principle	Advantages	Disadvantages	Common uses
AGID	Antigen and antibody diffuse through agar and form a visible precipitin line	Simple, inexpensive, no special equipment	Low sensitivity, slow (24–48 h), cross-reactivity	Bluetongue, EIA
Agglutination test	Antibodies cause visible clumping of antigen-coated particles	Rapid, easy, low cost	Qualitative/ semi-quantitative, false positives	Brucellosis, leptospirosis
VNT	Measures the ability of antibodies to neutralize live virus in cell culture	High specificity, functional (measures protective antibodies)	Time-consuming, requires live virus and BSL-2/3 lab	BVDV, IBR, Bluetongue serotyping
Indirect ELISA	Antigen-coated plate binds antibodies; enzyme-linked secondary antibody detects binding	High sensitivity/ specificity, quantitative, scalable	Requires equipment, may cross-react	BVDV, IBR, Johne's disease
cELISA	Antibody in the sample competes with the labeled antibody for antigen binding	High specificity, less affected by maternal antibodies	More complex, may be less sensitive than indirect ELISA	Bluetongue, FMD, BVDV

(Table 5.1). Until the past decade or so, agent detection has relied on the laboratory culture of invaders, primarily viruses and bacteria. With the advent of polymerase chain reaction (PCR) testing to detect invader DNA or RNA, much of the time and variability in culture-based methods has been alleviated. PCR testing, mostly so-called "real-time" or quantitative PCR testing, has replaced, or is replacing, culture methods in most diagnostic labs. Because of this focus on PCR testing, immunologic testing for exposure, usually by serologic testing, has become somewhat less commonly used; nevertheless, it can still be useful diagnostically, depending on the stage of an outbreak or the timing of sampling. As well, serological testing can be useful in assessing responses to vaccination.

What Are the Methodologies Used in Serological Testing? How Are Results Reported?

Agar Gel Immunodiffusion Test (AGID)

The AGID test was first developed in the 1950s and is still used today for some applications, notably for regulatory purposes to detect cattle that have been exposed to bluetongue virus. As well, an AGID test (*Coggins test*) is required for state diagnostic labs to diagnose equine infectious anemia (EIA) and has remained as one of the official laboratory tests for diagnosing EIA in approved U.S. Department of Agriculture laboratories.

The test is performed by pouring a thin layer of agar into a petri dish. Small wells are punched, usually with a central well surrounded by peripheral wells. Antigen is placed in the central well and sera in the surrounding wells, often alternating test sera with positive control serum. The antigen and antibody diffuse through the agar, and where they meet, if the antibody in the serum recognizes the antigen. A white line, the *precipitin line*, forms. This test is simple, inexpensive, does not require sophisticated equipment, and is useful for screening large numbers of animals. However, it is less sensitive than other serological tests and may not detect early infections, because it is not it does not detect IgM. That is because IgM, the predominant immunoglobulin early in infections, is large (pentameric) and diffuses poorly through the agar.

Agglutination Tests

Various agglutination tests are another example of "old, low-tech" methods that are still used. Generically, as the name implies, agglutination tests rely on the visual interpretation of an agglutination or clumping reaction between antibodies and, usually, particulate antigens. Currently, the most used example of an agglutination test is the *Rose Bengal plate test* globally performed for screening for antibodies to *Brucella abortus*. To do the test, a drop of test serum is applied to a white plastic or ceramic plate. An equal drop of Rose Bengal antigen is added. Rose Bengal antigen is inactivated *Brucella abortus* that has been stained with Rose Bengal dye and buffered to a low pH to help reduce non-specific reactions and increase the specificity of the test. The drops are mixed. A pink clump (agglutination) indicates the presence of antibodies against *Brucella*, and thus an active infection or previous exposure. The *Brucella Card Test* for serum and *Milk Ring Test* for milk are other examples of agglutination tests that have been used to test for antibodies to *B. abortus* in cattle.

Complement Fixation Tests (CFTs)

The CFT is another classical serological technique that is still used, primarily as a confirmatory test for other serological tests for *Brucella* spp., especially in regulatory and trade-related testing because of its *high specificity*. To do a CFT, test sera are mixed with an antigen, in this case, *Brucella abortus*. If a test serum contains antibodies against *Brucella*, immune complexes are formed. These are detected by adding complement, usually from guinea pig serum, which "fix" or consume the complement. This complement fixation can be visualized by the addition of anti-sheep antibody-coated sheep red blood cells. If the complement has been fixed or "used up" by the immune complexes, none will be there to lyse the red blood cells. Thus, the absence of *hemolysis* means a *positive test*. If there are no antibodies, and, therefore, no immune complexes, the complement causes *hemolysis*—interpreted as a *negative test*. In contrast to an AGID test, a CFT is very effective at detecting IgM because it is pentameric and highly efficient at fixing complement. This makes CFT particularly useful in detecting early infections. It can also detect IgG1, but not IgG2, again related to the respective complement-fixing ability of these isotypes.

Virus Neutralization Tests (VNTs)

Virus neutralization (VN) or *serum neutralization* tests were first developed in the late 1950s to study antibody responses to Eastern equine encephalitis virus in horses and, shortly thereafter, became central to the development of polio vaccines for humans. It has been adapted to a wide range of viruses in veterinary and human medicine and is still considered the gold standard for evaluating antibody responses and vaccine efficacy, mainly because it is a measure of a functional response. It is also called the *plaque reduction neutralization test (PRNT)* because it measures the ability of antibodies to reduce the number of *viral plaques* formed in a cell culture. A plaque is a visible focus of viral-induced damage or so-called *cytopathic effect (CPE)* in the monolayer of cultured cells. The nature of the CPE varies with the virus. Herpes viruses such as BHV-1 and bovine rotaviruses cause complete lysis or death of cells, and the plaques appear as clear areas. Viruses such as bovine respiratory syncytial virus (BRSV), bovine parainfluenza-3 virus (BPIV-3), and bovine coronavirus (BCoV) usually cause *syncytia*, which are rounded up and fused into multinucleated giant cells, which are also considered to be plaques. Non-cytopathic viruses, notably non-cytopathic strains of BVDV, do not cause visual damage, making interpretation of VN tests for these viruses more difficult. To perform a VN test, a known quantity of the virus is added to serial (usually twofold) dilutions of the test serum. The mixtures are incubated to allow any virus-specific antibodies in the serum to bind to and "neutralize" the virus. Although there are several means by which viruses can be neutralized or rendered incapable of infection, probably the most common mechanism measured in the VN test is simply the blocking of attachment to the cell. This is because antibodies bind to surface proteins that the virus uses to attach to host cell receptors, thereby blocking infection. After this initial incubation, the virus–serum mixtures are then added, usually in replicates of two or four, to well plates containing cultured monolayers of susceptible bovine cells, or susceptible cells from another species, notably Vero cells, which are monkey kidney cells that are susceptible to a wide range of viruses. The plates are incubated briefly to allow any non-neutralized virus to infect the cells. After this adsorption period, the cell monolayers are usually overlaid with a semi-solid medium, like agar or methylcellulose, to restrict cell-to-cell spread of the virus, ensuring that each non-neutralized particle forms a plaque, or localized focus of infection. The plates are then incubated for several days to allow plaques to develop, and then the monolayers are fixed and usually stained with crystal violet to make the plaques more visible. In the case of non-cytopathic viruses, immunohistochemical staining of the cellular monolayer can be done to visualize foci of infection. The *titer* is the last of the serum that neutralizes or prevents plaque formation. Alternatively, the titer can be reported as the dilution that prevents plaque formation in half of the wells in a replicate of two or four (*PRNT50*). Titers are reported either as that dilution or the reciprocal of that dilution. By convention, when *acute* (initial collection) and *convalescent* (at least 14 days after initial collection) sera are tested for evidence of a significant antibody response to an exposure to a microbe, natural or vaccinal, a fourfold increase in titer is indicative of *seroconversion*. The reason for this standard fourfold threshold is that it reduces the likelihood that the change is due to technical or biological variability in the assay and therefore represents a true response. When analyzing titers statistically, geometric (log-transformed) values should be used, hence the term *geometric mean titer*. For example, the geometric values for doubling (log_2) dilution titers 1:2, 1:4, 1:8, and 1:16 would be 1, 2, 3, and 4, respectively; the ones that should be used in any calculations.

Although the standard procedures for VN testing are long and well-established, there are several sources of *inter-laboratory* variability that make direct comparison of VN titers across different diagnostic laboratories unreliable at best. Labs may be using different isolates or strains of the same virus that may vary in their ability to grow in the cells being used, or in their susceptibility to being neutralized. For example, antibody responses measured to BVDV1 versus BVDV2 genotypes can differ dramatically, depending on exposure. Different cell lines, as well as different passages of the same cell line, can differ in their ability to support viral replication and plaque formation. For example, generally “older” cell lines, ones that have been passaged more times, are less susceptible to virus infection or produce less virus. Use of such a cell line versus a more susceptible cell line or primary culture could result in less virus growth, less plaques, and therefore a falsely inflated titer, because it could appear that less antibody is required to reduce plaque number. Variations in how sera are collected (e.g., hemolysis), stored, and thawed can impact on antibody activity. Multiple freeze-thaws, such as during shipment, should be avoided. Differences in assay conditions, such as incubation times, temperatures, and the use or not of different overlay media, can alter plaque development and resultant titers. Use of different definitions for neutralization endpoints (e.g., $PRNT_{50}$ vs. $PRNT_{90}$) can affect reported titers. Finally, there is the human factor. Manual steps such as preparation of serum dilutions and addition of the virus can introduce human error. Plaque counting is a somewhat subjective interpretation. Similar variations may inadvertently exist within the same laboratory over time, making it prudent to submit paired acute and convalescent sera simultaneously. Even with standardization and validation within each laboratory, unfortunately, inter-laboratory harmonization and consistent use of the same reference standards are lacking for tests for many viruses in veterinary medicine.

Enzyme-Linked Immunosorbent Assays (ELISAs)

Indirect ELISA

There are several types of ELISAs used for diagnostic purposes, but the most commonly used is the so-called *indirect ELISA* to measure antibodies. This test was first developed in the late 1970s to measure antibodies to human albumin, as a proof of principle to replace radioimmunoassays for safety concerns. In the early 1980s, ELISAs were first used in human medicine to measure antibodies against the human immunodeficiency virus and *Salmonella typhi*. At about the same time the test was first used in veterinary medicine to measure antibodies against canine adenovirus-2 in dogs. Since then, it has been applied to the measurement of antibodies against a wide range of pathogens in human and veterinary medicine. The reason it is called "indirect" is that the detection of the target, or *primary*, antibody is not done directly, but rather through an *enzyme-linked secondary*, antibody that binds to it. Usually, this antibody is against the species from which the sample was taken and is linked to *horseradish peroxidase* enzyme. Alternatively, enzyme-linked *Protein A* from *Staphylococcus aureus* and *Protein G* from *Streptococcus* spp. are used as secondary reagents. Both bind to the Fc portion of bovine immunoglobulin, but Protein G binds more strongly and should be used preferentially. Overall, this layered approach increases the sensitivity of the test, as well as its versatility, because the same secondary antibody can be used against primary antibodies with many different antigenic specificities.

To perform an indirect ELISA, an antigen is first coated to special "sticky" (adsorptive) polystyrene plates, usually 96-well microtiter plates. Non-specific binding sites are blocked, often with a diluted gelatin solution. A single dilution, often 1/50 of the test serum is added, and the plates are incubated. After washing the excess unbound antibody away, the enzyme-linked secondary reagent is added and allowed to react. After a final washing step, a substrate specific to the enzyme is added. Then the enzyme catalyzes a color change in the substrate; the more antibody bound by the antigen, the more intense the color in the well. The intensity of the color or optical density (OD) is measured on a spectrophotometer set at a wavelength that is optimal for the color of the reaction product, often 450 nm. In contrast to the VN test, results are reported as *units of activity*, not a titer. Units of activity are determined by a computerized comparison of the OD of a sample with a standard curve that is generated by preparing a series of dilutions of a positive control serum, which is run in parallel with the test samples. Ideally, a blank or negative control serum is also included in each assay. Diagnostic laboratories will often report units of activity and, in addition, whether they are to be considered low, medium, or high values (in their laboratory).

Competitive ELISA

Competitive ELISAs (cELISAs) to detect antibodies are a variation on the indirect ELISA theme. As the name implies, in this case, antibodies in a sample are measured by their ability to "compete" with an enzyme-labeled antibody, usually a monoclonal antibody, for the binding to an antigen. So, in cELISAs, the OD is *inversely proportional* to the amount of antibody in a sample. In other words, less color in a test well means more antibody because there is more antibody in the test serum to compete with the labeled antibody, and less of that can bind to the antigen.

Generally, cELISAs have higher sensitivity and specificity and are less prone to interference from non-specific binding than indirect ELISAs. They are particularly useful for measuring antibody responses to closely related antigens or microbes that differ in only a few epitopes, especially when testing complex mixtures like milk. For example, a cELISA can be used to differentiate responses to cytopathic versus non-cytopathic biotypes of BVDV by detecting antibodies to the nonstructural protein NS2–3, otherwise known as p80, which is only found in non-cytopathic variants of the virus. P80 is cleaved to separate NS2 and NS3 proteins in cytopathic variants that comprise by far the most vaccines. Applied to the diagnosis of BVDV infections, a cELISA would be particularly useful in differentiating infected from vaccinated animals and in screening bulk tank milk. cELISAs also have the advantage of being species-independent (they do use a species-specific secondary antibody), so they can be used to test a variety of ruminant species for antibodies to BVDV, or a closely related virus, for instance, potential reservoir cervids.

Indirect and cELISAs for antibody detection have several advantages over neutralization tests. They are generally faster because they do not require the growth of a virus or other microbe. Also, since usually only one dilution of serum is tested, they are suited to testing large numbers of samples concurrently. They also remove the subjectivity of interpreting CPE or plaque formation, since quantitation of colorimetric values is computerized. They are, at least in principle, easier to standardize. For these reasons, they are well-suited to diagnostic medicine and have replaced neutralization tests in many diagnostic laboratories. However, depending on how the antigen is prepared, ELISAs may not measure a functional antibody response. For example, measurement of antibodies to viral nuclear proteins or denatured envelope glycoproteins may not correlate with neutralizing activity. This makes ELISAs potentially less useful in assessing antibody responses to vaccination unless direct comparisons between ELISAs and VNs have been made.

How Can ELISAs Be Used to Detect Antigen (Versus Antibody)?

Antigen Capture ELISA (ACE)

ACE or "*sandwich*" *ELISAs* are so named because an antigen is captured or sandwiched between two antibodies, a capture antibody, and a detection antibody. The way this test is done is to immobilize the capture antibody on a microplate well or membrane (especially for in-clinic applications). Non-specific binding sites are blocked, and the test sample is added. After a washing step, an enzyme-linked antibody is added, followed by a color-producing substrate. In these tests, usually, the capture antibody is a polyclonal antiserum because it can recognize multiple epitopes on the target antigen, whereas the detection antibody is usually a monoclonal antibody that binds one specific epitope. The use of a monoclonal antibody increases the specificity of the test and reduces background staining, which eases interpretation.

Although PCR is replacing culturing and other methods of antigen detection in diagnostic medicine, ACEs are still used in some applications, notably for commonly used in-clinic tests for Feline leukemia virus and canine parvovirus. Nevertheless, there have been two main applications of this technology in bovine medicine, for the diagnosis of BVDV and *Mycobacteria* spp. infections, both of which are performed in laboratory settings. For BVDV, there have been two ACEs with different target antigens, both of which are aimed primarily at detecting PI cattle, usually calves. One detects the *envelope ribonuclease activity (Erns) glycoprotein of the virus* that is present in both cytopathic and noncytopathic biotypes of the virus. It is stable, secreted, and not neutralized by antibody, making it a good target. Although this ACE can be used on serum samples, it has been more commonly used on ear notch biopsies, which are soaked in a lysis buffer to extract the BVDV protein. Compared to PCR on blood, it has the advantage of only requiring one test, since if a calf has detectable BVDV antigen in the skin, it is almost certainly PI. In contrast, a single detection of BVDV RNA (by reverse-transcriptase PCR) in the blood could indicate a resolvable acute infection, necessitating a re-test. There is also a less-used ACE for BVDV p80. This is primarily applied to blood (serum) samples and can differentiate cattle vaccinated with marker (DIVA) vaccines versus infected individuals.

Another ACE has application in the diagnosis of *Mycobacterium bovis* infections. It does not detect the bacteria, but rather a *CMI* (interferon-γ) *response* to the bacteria. The test involves stimulating whole blood with purified protein derivative from *M. bovis*, then measuring the release of IFN-γ into the plasma using an ACE. This test is usually used as a supplementary or confirmatory test for the tuberculin skin (fold) test. It has also been used in research to assess a CMI (Th1-like) response to a variety of antigens, for instance.

Your Case

You are contemplating using a new injectable combination viral vaccine for the prevention of bovine respiratory disease. To compare the vaccine you are currently using with the new one in your practice population, you decide to measure antibody responses to the BHV-1 component of the vaccines. To do this in one of your client's cow–calf herds, the client and you randomly select 50 weanling Angus calves that are co-housed in the same pasture—half randomly receive the current vaccine, and half randomly receive the new vaccine. Before vaccination, you collect blood, harvest serum ("acute" sample), and send it off to the diagnostic lab for the determination of neutralizing antibody titers. About a week later, you get the results. Eye-balling them, the average VN titer looks to be about 1:8 in both groups. About 2 weeks later, you run the calves through the chute again, collect another batch of serum ("convalescent" sample), and submit it. When you get results this time, again, quickly running the numbers in your head, calves that received the "old" vaccine seem to have titers averaging 1:32; whereas the calves that received the new vaccine had titers that averaged 1:16.

Questions for You

1. Would an apparent twofold difference in response to the two vaccines be indicative of a significant difference in responses to the two vaccines?
2. If you decide, for financial purposes, to change diagnostic laboratories, should you compare the VN results from two different laboratories, assuming that they use the same standard procedures: why or why not? What about assays conducted on two different days in the same laboratory?
3. Some diagnostic laboratories use VNTs to quantitate virus-specific antibody responses, and others use ELISA tests. What is the difference in the way the tests are done and the way the results are determined and reported?

Additional Readings

1. Tizard I. Immunodiagnostic techniques. In: Veterinary immunology. 10th ed. Elsevier; 2018. p. 472–87.
2. Hayrapetyan H, Tran T, Tellez-Corrales E, Madiraju C. Enzyme-linked immunosorbent assay: types and applications. Methods Mol Biol. 2023;2612:1–17. https://doi.org/10.1007/978-1-0716-2903-1_1.
3. Woolums AR. Serology in bovine infectious disease diagnosis. Vet Clin Food Pract. 2023;39:141–55.

Part II

The Immune System in Cattle

6 Mucosal Immunity

Abstract

The mucosal immune system is one of the most complicated systems in the body. The system must not only limit and remove virulent microorganisms but also maintain the delicate balance of the microbiome found in the various mucosal compartments. When in proper balance, the local immune system not only improves health but also positively impacts many body functions, improving production parameters. The first line of interaction in the mucosal immune system is the innate system, which comprises mechanical and chemical barriers, as well as cells of the innate system.

Keywords

Mucosal immunology · Microbiome · Dendritic cells · Regulatory T cells (Tregs) · $\gamma\delta +$ T cells · Gamma delta T cells · Barrier defenses · Innate immunity

Key Concepts

- The mucosal immune system is the largest immune system in the body and is comprised of several different specialized systems.
- Since the local immune system interacts with the microbiome, its primary job is to monitor and maintain microflora balance.
- The local immune system must also be able to recognize and respond to pathogenic invaders and correct microflora imbalances.

J. Ellis, V. Cortese, *Practical Bovine Immunology*,
https://doi.org/10.1007/978-3-032-15031-8_6

What Is the Mucosal Immune System?

The *mucosal immune system* is responsible for monitoring and protecting the body against exposures that occur at *mucosal membranes* of the intestines, the urogenital (reproductive) tract, including the mammary gland, the eye, and the respiratory system [1–4]. The mucous membranes are located near the surfaces where most pathogens invade; thus, they are in constant exposure to microorganisms, food, allergens, and other antigens [1–4]. Thus, the mucosal immune system is a first line of defense against foreign antigens. The mucosal immune system has four primary functions:

A. Protect the body from organisms and allergens encountered at the mucosal surfaces.
B. Monitor and react to antigens that the system is being exposed to.
C. Maintain tolerance and control levels of the biome microflora.
D. Trap and remove toxins, pollutants, and allergens.

Recent studies indicate that there are three distinct mucosal immune systems based on T cell/B cell address in interactions that drive homing patterns after stimulation. These include respiratory and reproductive (RESP-RT), gastrointestinal (GI), and ocular mucosal immune systems [5–10]. While studies listed above show separation between the RESP-RT and GI mucosal immune systems, intranasal vaccination with an adenovirus stimulated both the RESP-RT and GI mucosal immune systems. It is not clear if some of the intranasal vaccine drained to the oral cavity, activating the GI mucosal immune system, or if some cross communication may occur [5].

The mucosal immune system involves physical barriers and components of the innate and adaptive immune system that are located near the epithelial surfaces.

How Does the Mucosal Immune System Function?

The first line of defense of the mucosal immune system consist of the *epithelial cells and mucus* on the cell surface that form a tight barrier [11, 12]. The integrity of the epithelial-mucus surface physically stops pathogens from entering the body [11]. *The submucosal gland epithelial cells* (mucous, serous cells, and secretory goblet cells), besides manufacturing mucus, also secrete electrolytes, antimicrobial, and anti-inflammatory proteins onto mucosal surfaces [11–13]. *Mucins* shield the mucosa from attack by the mucosa, thereby limiting the immunogenicity of incoming antigens. This prevents many unneeded inflammatory responses by dendritic cells (DCs) [11–13]. While the muco-epithelial barrier is similar throughout the mucosal system, there are slight differences between the respiratory, gastrointestinal, and reproductive systems, which are discussed below.

The respiratory tract barrier is augmented by cilia that form the mucociliary escalator that removes particles and pathogens by the mechanical actions of cilia supplemented by coughing [13]. The nasal mucosa also plays an important role in warming and humidifying incoming air, protecting the integrity of the mucociliary lining of the airways [14–17]. The epithelial surface liquid comprises two layers: a periciliary layer that is a more liquid layer close to the cell surface and a gel/mucus layer at the interface of the airway lumen [18]. One study of healthy animals showed that the mucociliary apparatus could clear greater than 90% of aerosolized bacteria within 4 h of administration [19]. Only particles smaller than 5–6 μm can bypass a healthy, intact mucociliary system [20, 21]; however, this system can be disrupted by a myriad of infections and stresses [14–17].

While the barrier system of the gastrointestinal tract does not have the cilia of the respiratory barrier, it is comprised of several areas that have different methods of providing a barrier (more than 90% of potential pathogens are GI associated) [4] and maintain balance with the commensal bacteria and microbiome. The oral mucosa provides first-line protection against potential pathogens, exogenous chemicals, airborne allergens, and so on [22, 23]. The oral cavity is inhabited by a wide spectrum of microbial species but the integrity of its mucosal surface provides a mechanical barrier so that it is impermeable to most microorganisms and their penetration into tissues. This is further augmented by the rapid turnover and renewal of the oral epithelium. The oral epithelium is differentiated into keratinized as well as non-keratinized cells, and the places subjected to mechanical irritation while chewing have a keratin protective layer. The oral mucosa also reduces the colonization of microorganisms with the secretion of various types of cytokines and antimicrobial proteins such as defensins [22, 23]. As a chemical barrier, saliva (high content of IgA, mucins, and antimicrobial peptides (AMPs)) plays a very important role in those secretions [24].

The lower gastrointestinal mucosal barrier selectively allows the absorption of nutrients, prevents pathogen invasion, prevents loss of water and electrolytes, and forms and removes waste [24]. In addition, the intestinal epithelium is the barrier portion of the largest immune organ in cattle [4, 25]. The intestinal epithelium is composed of multiple cell types that form highly organized villi and are embedded within the epithelial layer. This includes Paneth cells, Goblet cells, tuft cells, enteroendocrine cells, and M cells. These cells release AMPs, other cytokines and hormones, secrete mucin, and participate in antigen sampling and presentation [4, 24–29].

The purpose of the *female reproductive tract (FRT)* is to allow fertilization, implantation, and development of the fetus [30, 31]. The vagina and exterior portion of the cervix are populated by commensal flora. The vaginal immune system allows the growth of beneficial microbes, samples microflora, and prevents pathogen buildup [4, 25, 30, 31]. The cervix prevents upward movement of microbes into the uterus but allows the passage of sperm. The FRT immune system in the uterus develops specific tolerance of immunologically distinct sperm and the fetus [30, 31]. Unique to the reproductive tract immune system is the impact of hormones, reproduction, pregnancy, and post-partum uterine involution [30, 32]. Cervico-vaginal mucus composition, viscosity, and volume and composition of microbial population vary during the reproductive cycle [33]. During pregnancy, the cervix is filled with a thick secretion (cervical plug) that prevents infections from entering through the vagina. The physical barrier of the FRT tract, similar to the respiratory and gastrointestinal barriers, is comprised of a muco-epithelial layer (stratified squamous epithelium of the vagina) [31, 34]. AMPs and mucosal glycoproteins also cover the mucosa to neutralize bacteria and prevent them from reaching the epithelium (β-defensins, lingual AMP, and tracheal AMP) [31, 34–36].

The mammary gland, particularly in dairy cattle, has its own challenges. The teat canal is the primary barrier defense against mastitis. A *keratin plug* seals the canal between milkings and during the dry period [37, 38]. The stratified epithelial lining of the canal produces this plug, and it provides a physical barrier that prevents bacteria from moving into the mammary gland. Keratin also has some microbiocidal activity against mastitis causing pathogens [37, 38]. Milking flushes out the keratin plug and any residual microbes in the canal and bathes the teat cistern and canal with antimicrobials. The teat end contains sphincter muscles that maintain tight closure between milkings. In contrast to the respiratory and gastrointestinal tracts, the teat canal barrier maintains the aseptic nature of the mammary gland [37, 38]. Thus, the mammary epithelium is only stimulated by bacteria when mastitis occurs.

Active Immunity of the Mucosal Tissues

While the barriers of the mucosal system are considered passive, it is obvious that they are active in providing first-line defenses of the mucosal surfaces. However, since they do not require cells of the immune system to provide this protection, it is considered immunologically passive. The active mucosal immune system, like the systemic immune system, comprises both the innate and adaptive components of the immune system [36–39]. This is a rather local but specialized version of the immune system and is well interlinked with the lymphatic system, and thus it is known as mucosa-associated lymphatic tissue or, in a more functional sense, the mucosal immune system. There are various subsets of this broad term, including gut-associated lymphatic tissue, bronchus-associated lymphatic tissue, and nasal-associated lymphatic tissue. The active mucosal immune system has two parts: the innate system and the adaptive system. The innate system comprises various recognition molecules and natural killer cells, while the adaptive system comprises various antigen-presenting cells and the T and B lymphocytes.

What Comprises the Mucosal Innate Immune System?

The mucosal innate immune system acts not only as an immunological barrier but also plays the primary role in sensing and eliminating pathogens and maintaining the balance required by the various microflora of the mucosal biomes. As more is learned about the cells of the innate immune system, some immunologists are including them in the adaptive rather than the innate immune system. While many of the cells are similar in the systemic and local innate immune systems (neutrophils, natural killer cells, and macrophages) [39–41] (see Chap. 2), the function of the local antigen presentation is different from systemic macrophage presentation and is assisted by potent antigen-presenting cells named *DCs*.

Rather than a single cell type, *bovine DCs* comprise subsets of different (phenotypes) DCs with different biological properties [42, 43]. Considered to be the only cells able to present antigen to naive T cells and initiate primary immune responses [42], DCs are found on mucosal surfaces and recognize pathogen-associated microbial patterns (PAMPs) (see Chap. 2) using pattern recognition receptors (PRR), (similar to toll cell-like receptors) in both infected cells and pathogens [36–43]. On finding an infected cell, pattern recognition receptors induce the secretion of interferons and DC-activating cytokines. This is followed by major histocompatibility complex (MHC) Class I presentation. If PAMPs are encountered, costimulatory molecules are released, PRRs recognize the pathogen, and the pathogen and PRR are processed via phagocytosis. Antigen presentation occurs with the MHC Class II pathway [43–45].

Another critical feature of this system is the ability to differentiate, via pattern recognition receptors, between pathogenic and nonpathogenic microflora [44, 46], maintaining the microbiome environment on mucosal surfaces. DCs can also secrete proteins that prevent damage from proinflammatory cytokines on mucosal surfaces [47] and release CD14 molecules that bind to lipopolysaccharides and regulate interactions between the microbiota and the mucosa [45].

What About the Adaptive Mucosal Immune System?

The continuous exposure of the mucosa to external antigens and microbiota requires that majority of the body's adaptive immune cells are involved with mucosal immunity. "For example, approximately 3/4 of all lymphocytes are found in the mucous membranes" [38]. The basic adaptive immune responses of the mucosal immune response are similar to the systemic immune responses, with several notable differences.

While mucosal epithelial cells are critical for mucosal functions and protection, they also transport immunoglobulins produced by plasma cells to mucosal surfaces [48]. While in low levels in the serum, the primary secretory antibody in mammals is IgA. Both nasal-associated lymphoid tissue and Peyer's patches generate IgA and IgG1 antibodies (as well as low levels of IgM and IgG2) [44]. *Secretory IgA (sIgA)* is a diameric protein composed of two IgA units (two heavy and two light chains), a joining J peptide chain, and a non-immunoglobulin moiety called the secretory component [49]. However, IgG1 is also a secretory immunoglobulin in ruminants [50–52] and is found on most mucosal surfaces. The adaptive mucosal immune system is involved in maintaining mucosal homeostasis through a mechanism of immune exclusion mediated by secretory antibodies that inhibit the penetration of invasive pathogens into the body's tissues and prevent the penetration of potentially dangerous exogenous proteins [53]. It is also important to note that IgG1, not IgA, is the predominant colostral antibody in cattle [54].

While there are large number of B lymphocytes (and plasma cells) associated with the mucosal immune system, intraepithelial T lymphocytes comprise over 50% of the total T lymphocytes in cattle [55, 56]. Similar to other cells of the mucosal immune system, T cells patrol the mucosa, defending against pathogen invasion and maintaining homeostasis [57]. The mucosal-associated T lymphoid cells are composed primarily of regulatory T cells (Tregs), CD8+, and γδ + T cells [36–38, 48, 55, 56].

Tregs can cause immunosuppressive (primarily through anti-inflammatory cytokines) mechanisms to prevent local and peripheral hypersensitivity to microbiome-derived antigens [47, 58, 59]. Tregs are also involved in fetal–maternal tolerance during pregnancy [59]. One important difference between systemic and mucosal T cells is that mucosal-associated T cells do not require activation like classic T cells. This facilitates quicker removal of pathogens when these T cells recognize an antigen [48].

How Does the Neonatal Mucosal Immune System Develop?

At birth, neonates possess immature mucosal immune systems [38, 59–61]. The development of the mucosal immune system is influenced by numerous factors. These include colostrum (antibodies, white blood cells, cytokines, and other hormones), nutrition, and the developing microbiome [38, 60, 62–65]. The mucosal barriers of the in-utero calf have very limited exposure to outside influences; after birth, they are exposed to tremendous environmental, nutritional, and microbial exposures. The microbiome develops in sync with the development of the mucosal immune system [53, 60, 63, 65–67]. Timing and type of interactions between these two systems determine much of the long-term immune characteristics of these mucosal immune systems, that is, their susceptibility to infections and inflammatory diseases. As an example, mucosal B cell lineage is regulated by signals from the microbiome, affecting the intestinal immunoglobulin repertoire [53]. Maturation of the calves' mucosal immune system is complete by approximately 180 days of age [60, 65, 68].

What About Vaccines Delivered to the Mucosa in Cattle?

Mucosal delivered vaccines have been utilized in bovine vaccine programs for over 50 years [69, 70]. Mucosal vaccination can stimulate the immune system in different ways from systemic vaccination [68, 71–74] and is often included in vaccination programs that also include systemic vaccination. Most mucosal vaccines are modified live, but inactivated bacterins are also available. Intranasal and oral administration have been the favored routes, although rectal and vaginal delivery have also been explored [75–77].

Conclusion

The mucosal immune system comprises the largest and most complex system in the body. This is required to balance the monitoring and preserving of the beneficial microflora, assisting in body functions, and removing pathogens. When properly functioning, growth, health, and performance can be enhanced. Conversely, if the local immune system is damaged or inadequate, health is severely impacted, and death can often occur.

Your Case

History

A backgrounding facility in Virginia buys moderate to high-risk, lightweight (350–400 pounds) calves out of the Southeast. The calves are of mixed origin and a combination of steers and bulls. The calves are backgrounded for 60–90 days before being sold to a feedlot in Kansas. Backgrounding includes vaccination with a modified live viral vaccine containing BRSV, BHV-1, BPI3, and BVDV types 1 and 2 with *Mannheimia hemolytica* bacterin, seven-strain clostridia vaccine, and *Histophilus somnus* vaccination 12–24 h after arrival. The vaccines are repeated, bulls are surgically castrated, and calves are implanted 10–14 days after arrival. Death loss ranges between 5% and 11%.

Current Situation

One hundred, 300–350-pound bull calves were bought from an auction barn in southern Georgia. Calves came from various sources, were freshly weaned, and had unknown vaccination histories. Calves arrived in a thunderstorm and were deemed to be high risk based on history and appearance on arrival. They were sorted into three pens with a capacity of 40 calves (400-pound calves, based on bunk space). Due to the forecast of continued inclement weather, it was decided to postpone the initial vaccination until the weather broke (predicted at 72 h after arrival).

Situation

Approximately 48 h after arrival, 10 calves across the three pens were anorexic, depressed, and breathing hard. Upon examination, the calves had temperatures of 105–107 °F, muco-purulent nasal discharge, coughing, and increased respiratory sounds. A presumptive diagnosis of pneumonia was made, and the calves were moved to a treatment pen and treated with a long-acting cephalosporin. The following day, two of the treated calves had died, and two more were recumbent. The remaining six calves were not improving, and six more calves, with similar symptoms, were taken to the sick pen for examination and treatment.

Necropsy Findings

You euthanized the two recumbent calves, and four necropsies were performed. Three of the four calves had some nasal ulcers, and one calf had a few small oral ulcers. The calves were thin and dehydrated, with necrotizing laryngotracheitis (Fig. 6.1), often accompanied by secondary bacterial pneumonia. The trachea (4/4) and larynx (2/4) had extensive necrotic damage and were malodorous with a pseudo-membrane. Cranioventral lung lobes were reddish-purple and slightly edematous and emphysematous. Some lung consolidation was noted.

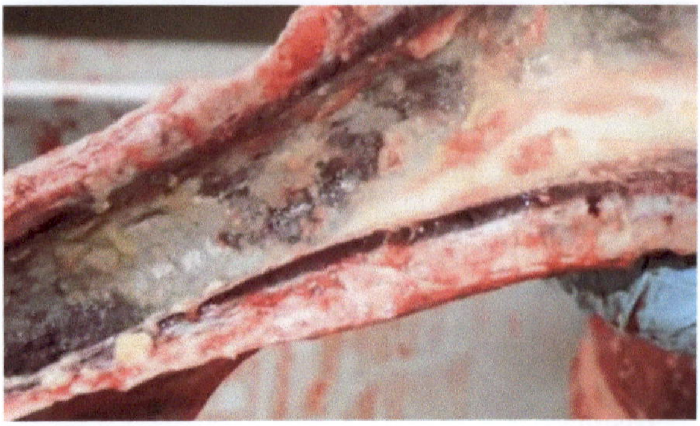

Fig. 6.1 Photograph of larynx and trachea from necropsied calf

Questions for You

1. Based on history and necropsy, what is your presumptive diagnosis?
2. Based on your diagnosis, how do you proceed?
3. How do you explain the rapid and high mortality rate in the infected cattle?

Additional Readings

1. Zheng D, Liwinski T, Elinav E. Interaction between microbiota and immunity in health and disease. Cell Res. 2020;30(6):492–506. https://doi.org/10.1038/s41422-020-0332-7. PMC 7264227. PMID 32433595.
2. Csencsits KL, Walters N, Pascual DW. Cutting edge: dichotomy of homing receptor dependence by mucosal effector B cells: alpha(E) versus L-selectin. J Immunol. 2001;167(5):2441–5.
3. Abitorabi MA, Mackay CR, Jerome EH, Osorio O, Butcher EC, Erle DJ. Differential expression of homing molecules on recirculating lymphocytes from sheep gut, peripheral, and lung lymph. J Immunol. 1996;156:3111.
4. Csencsits KL, Jutila MA, Pascual DW. Nasal-associated lymphoid tissue: phenotypic and functional evidence for the primary role of peripheral node addressin in naive lymphocyte adhesion to high endothelial venules in a mucosal site. J Immunol. 1999;163:1382.
5. Perry LL, Feilzer K, Portis JL, Caldwell HD. Distinct homing pathways direct T lymphocytes to the genital and intestinal mucosae in chlamydia infected mice. J Immunol. 1998;160:2905.
6. Pascual D, White MD, Larson T, Walters N. Impaired mucosal immunity in L-selectin-deficient mice orally immunized with a Salmonella vaccine vector. J Immunol. 2001;167:407.
7. de Paiva CS, St Leger AJ, Caspi RR. Mucosal immunology of the ocular surface. Mucosal Immunol. 2022;15(6):1143–57. https://doi.org/10.1038/s41385-022-00551-6. Epub 2022 Aug 24. PMID: 36002743; PMCID: PMC9400566.
8. Okumura R, Takeda K. Maintenance of intestinal homeostasis by mucosal barriers. Inflamm Regen. 2018;38(1):5. https://doi.org/10.1186/s41232-018-0063-z. PMC 5879757. PMID 29619131.
9. Shan M, Gentile M, Yeiser JR, Walland AC, Bornstein VU, Chen K, He B, Cassis L, Bigas A, Cols M, Comerma L, Huang B, Blander JM, Xiong H, Mayer L, Berin C, Augenlicht LH, Velcich A, Cerutti A. Mucus enhances gut homeostasis and oral tolerance by delivering immunoregulatory signals. Science. 2013;342(6157):447–53. https://doi.org/10.1126/science.1237910. Epub 2013 Sep 26. PMID: 24072822; PMCID: PMC4005805.

10. Whitsett JA. Airway epithelial differentiation and Mucociliary clearance. Ann Am Thorac Soc. 2018;15(Suppl 3):S143–8. https://doi.org/10.1513/AnnalsATS.201802-128AW. PMID: 30431340; PMCID: PMC6322033.
11. Harkema JR, Carey SA, Wagner JG. The nose revisited: a brief review of the comparative structure, function, and Toxicologic pathology of the nasal epithelium. Toxicol Pathol. 2006;34(3):252–69. https://doi.org/10.1080/01926230600713475.
12. Caswell JL. Failure of respiratory defenses in the pathogenesis of bacterial pneumonia of cattle. Vet Pathol. 2014;51(2):393–409. https://doi.org/10.1177/0300985813502821.
13. Diesel DA, Lebel JL, Tucker A. Pulmonary particle deposition and airway mucociliary clearance in cold-exposed calves. Am J Vet Res. 1991;52(10):1665–71.
14. Jones CD. Proliferation of Pasteurella haemolytica in the calf respiratory tract after an abrupt change in climate. Res Vet Sci. 1987;42(2):179–86.
15. Ackermann MR, Derscheid R, Roth JA. Innate immunology of bovine respiratory disease. Vet Clin North Am Food Anim Pract. 2010;26(2):215–28. https://doi.org/10.1016/j.cvfa.2010.03.001. Epub 2010 May 14. PMID: 20619180; PMCID: PMC2904317.
16. Lopez A, Maxie MG, Savan M. The pulmonary clearance of Pasteurella haemolytica in calves infected with bovine virus diarrhea or Mycoplasma bovis. Can J Comp Med. 1982;46:302–6.
17. Ferin J. Pulmonary retention and clearance of particles. Toxicol Lett. 1994;72(1–3):121–5. https://doi.org/10.1016/0378-4274(94)90018-3.
18. Perino LJ. Immunology and prevention of bovine respiratory disease in bovine respiratory disease, veterinary learning systems. 1996;
19. Ptasiewicz M, Grywalska E, Mertowska P, Korona-Głowniak I, Poniewierska-Baran A, Niedźwiedzka-Rystwej P, Chałas R. Armed to the teeth-the Oral mucosa immunity system and microbiota. Int J Mol Sci. 2022;23(2):882. https://doi.org/10.3390/ijms23020882. PMID: 35055069; PMCID: PMC8776045.
20. Şenel S. An overview of physical, microbiological and immune barriers of Oral mucosa. Int J Mol Sci. 2021;22(15):7821. https://doi.org/10.3390/ijms22157821. PMID: 34360589; PMCID: PMC8346143.
21. Suárez LJ, Arboleda S, Angelov N, Arce RM. Oral versus gastrointestinal Mucosal immune niches in homeostasis and Allostasis. Front Immunol. 2021;12:705206. https://doi.org/10.3389/fimmu.2021.705206. PMID: 34290715; PMCID: PMC8287884.
22. Chase CCL. Enteric immunity: happy gut, healthy animal. Vet Clin North Am Food Anim Pract. 2018;34(1):1–18. https://doi.org/10.1016/j.cvfa.2017.10.006. PMID: 29421027; PMCID: PMC7125775.
23. Allaire JM, Crowley SM, Law HT, Chang SY, Ko HJ, Vallance BA. The intestinal epithelium: central coordinator of Mucosal immunity. Trends Immunol. 2018;39(9):677–96. https://doi.org/10.1016/j.it.2018.04.002.
24. Kuper CF. Histopathology of mucosa-associated lymphoid tissue. Toxicol Pathol. 2006;34(5):609–15. https://doi.org/10.1080/01926230600867735.
25. Shi J. Defensins and Paneth cells in inflammatory bowel disease. Inflamm Bowel Dis. 2007;13(10):1284–92. https://doi.org/10.1002/ibd.20197.
26. Ma J, Rubin BK, Voynow JA. Mucins, mucus, and goblet cells. Chest. 2018;154(1):169–76. https://doi.org/10.1016/j.chest.2017.11.008. Epub 2017 Nov 21. PMID: 29170036.
27. Monin L, Whettlock EM, Male V. Immune responses in the human female reproductive tract. Immunology. 2020;160(2):106–15. https://doi.org/10.1111/imm.13136. Epub 2019 Nov 11. PMID: 31630394; PMCID: PMC7218661.
28. Sheldon IM, Cronin JG, Healey GD, Gabler C, Heuwieser W, Streyl D, Bromfield JJ, Miyamoto A, Fergani C, Dobson H. Innate immunity and inflammation of the bovine female reproductive tract in health and disease. Reproduction. 2014;148(3):R41–51. https://doi.org/10.1530/REP-14-0163. Epub 2014 Jun 2. PMID: 24890752.
29. Collins MK, McCutcheon CR, Petroff MG. Impact of estrogen and progesterone on immune cells and host–pathogen interactions in the lower female reproductive tract. J Immunol. 2022;209(8):1437–49. https://doi.org/10.4049/jimmunol.2200454.

30. Srinivasan M, Adnane M, Archunan G. Significance of cervico-vaginal microbes in bovine reproduction and pheromone production – a hypothetical review. Res Vet Sci. 2021;135:66–71. https://doi.org/10.1016/j.rvsc.2021.01.003. ISSN 0034-5288.
31. Davies D, Meade KG, Herath S, Eckersall PD, Gonzalez D, White JO, Conlan RS, O'Farrelly C, Sheldon IM. Toll-like receptor and antimicrobial peptide expression in the bovine endometrium. Reprod Biol Endocrinol. 2008;6(1):53. https://doi.org/10.1186/1477-7827-6-53.
32. DeSouza MM, Surveyor GA, Price RE, Julian J, Kardon R, Zhou X, Gendler S, Hilkens J, Carson DD. MUC1/episialin: a critical barrier in the female reproductive tract. J Reprod Immunol. 1999;45:127–58. https://doi.org/10.1016/S0165-0378(99)00046-7.
33. Chapwanya A, Meade KG, Doherty ML, Callanan JJ, O'Farrelly C. Endometrial epithelial cells are potent producers of tracheal antimicrobial peptide and serum amyloid A3 gene expression in response to E. coli stimulation. Vet Immunol Immunopathol. 2013;151:157–62. https://doi.org/10.1016/j.vetimm.2012.09.042.
34. Rainard P, Riollet C. Innate immunity of the bovine mammary gland. Vet Res. 2006;37:369–400. https://doi.org/10.1051/vetres:2006007.
35. Craven N, Williams MR. Defences of the bovine mammary gland against infection and prospects for their enhancement. Vet Immunol Immunopathol. 1985;10:71–127.
36. McGhee JR, Fujihashi K. Inside the mucosal immune system. PLoS Biol. 2012;10(9):e1001397. https://doi.org/10.1371/journal.pbio.1001397. Epub 2012 Sep 25. PMID: 23049482; PMCID: PMC3457930.
37. Kiyono H, Kweon MN, Hiroi T, Takahashi I. The mucosal immune system: from specialized immune defense to inflammation and allergy. Acta Odontol Scand. 2001;59(3):145–53. https://doi.org/10.1080/000163501750266738.
38. Chase C, Kaushik RS. System Mucosal immune of cattle: all immune responses begin here. Vet Clin North Am Food Anim Pract. 2019;35(3):431–45.
39. Dwivedy A, Aich P. Importance of innate mucosal immunity and the promises it holds. Int J Gen Med. 2011;4:299–311. https://doi.org/10.2147/IJGM.S17525. PMID: 21556316; PMCID: PMC3085239.
40. Nochi T, Kiyono H. Innate immunity in the mucosal immune system. Curr Pharm Des. 2006;12(32):4203–13. https://doi.org/10.2174/138161206778743457.
41. Medzhitov R, Janeway C Jr. Innate immune recognition: mechanisms and pathways. Immunol Rev. 2000;173:89–97. https://doi.org/10.1034/j.1600-065x.2000.917309.x.
42. Howard CJ, Brooke GP, Werling D, Sopp P, Hope JC, Parsons KR, Collins RA. Dendritic cells in cattle: phenotype and function. Vet Immunol Immunopathol. 1999;72(1–2):119–24. https://doi.org/10.1016/s0165-2427(99)00124-5.
43. Shortman K, Caux C. Dendritic cell development: multiple pathways to nature's adjuvants. Stem Cells. 1997;15(6):409–19. https://doi.org/10.1002/stem.150409.
44. Sonnenberg GF, Hepworth MR. Functional interactions between innate lymphoid cells and adaptive immunity. Nat Rev Immunol. 2019;19(10):599–613. https://doi.org/10.1038/s41577-019-0194-8. PMC 6982279. PMID 31350531.
45. Stagg AJ. Intestinal dendritic cells in health and gut inflammation. Front Immunol. 2018;9:2883. https://doi.org/10.3389/fimmu.2018.02883. PMC 6291504. PMID 30574151.
46. Traxinger BR, Richert-Spuhler LE, Lund JM. Mucosal tissue regulatory T cells are integral in balancing immunity and tolerance at portals of antigen entry. Mucosal Immunol. 2021;15(3):398–407. https://doi.org/10.1038/s41385-021-00471-x. PMC 8628059. PMID 34845322.
47. Dillon A, Lo DD. M cells: intelligent engineering of Mucosal immune surveillance. Front Immunol. 2019;10:1499. https://doi.org/10.3389/fimmu.2019.01499. PMC 6614372. PMID 31312204.
48. Mörbe UM, Jørgensen PB, Fenton TM, von Burg N, Riis LB, Spencer J, Agace WW. Human gut-associated lymphoid tissues (GALT); diversity, structure, and function. Mucosal Immunol. 2021;14(4):793–802. https://doi.org/10.1038/s41385-021-00389-4. PMID 33753873. S2CID 232322692.

49. Li Y, Jin L, Chen T. The effects of secretory IgA in the Mucosal immune system. Biomed Res Int. 2020;3:2032057. https://doi.org/10.1155/2020/2032057. PMID: 31998782; PMCID: PMC6970489.
50. Duncan JR, Wilkie BN, Hiestand F, Winter AJ. The serum and secretory immunoglobulins of cattle: characterization and quantitation. J Immunol. 1972;108(4):965–76. https://doi.org/10.4049/jimmunol.108.4.965.
51. Cripps A, Husband AJ, Lascelles AK. The origin of immunoglobulins in intestinal secretion of sheep. Aust J Exp Biol Med Sci. 1974;52:711–6. https://doi.org/10.1038/icb.1974.70.
52. Lee CW, Shewen PE. Evidence of bovine immunoglobulin G1 (IgG1) protease activity in partially purified culture supernate of Pasteurella haemolytica A1. Can J Vet Res. 1996;60(2):127–32. PMID: 8785718; PMCID: PMC1263818
53. Wesemann DR, Portuguese AJ, Meyers RM, Gallagher MP, Cluff-Jones K, Magee JM, Rohit Panchakshari RA, Rodig SJ, Kepler TB, Alt FW. Microbial colonization influences early B-lineage development in the gut lamina propria. Nature. 2013;501(7465):112–5. https://doi.org/10.1038/nature12496. PMC 3807868. PMID 23965619.
54. Butler JE. Bovine Immunoglobulins: a Review. J Dairy Sci. 1969;52(12):1895–909.
55. Hada A, Li L, Kandel A, Jin Y, Xiao Z. Characterization of bovine intraepithelial T lymphocytes in the gut. Pathogens. 2023;12(9):1173. https://doi.org/10.3390/pathogens12091173.
56. Guzman E, Price S, Poulsom h, Hope J. Bovine γδ T cells: cells with multiple functions and important roles in immunity. Vet Immunol Immunopathol. 2012;148(1–2):161–7. https://doi.org/10.1016/j.vetimm.2011.03.013. ISSN 0165-2427.
57. Tordesillas L, Berin MC. Mechanisms of Oral tolerance. Clin Rev Allergy Immunol. 2018;55(2):107–17. https://doi.org/10.1007/s12016-018-8680-5. PMC 6110983. PMID 29488131.
58. Pandit A, Shah SM, Shah RA, Qureshi S, Sethi RS, Bhat F, Malik A, Parray O, Yaqoob H, Saleem M. Regulatory T cells in bovine fertility: current understanding and future prospects. Anim Reprod Sci. 2025;272:107655. https://doi.org/10.1016/j.anireprosci.2024.107655. ISSN 0378-4320.
59. Capozzo AV, Cuberos L, Levine MM, Pasetti MF. Mucosally delivered Salmonella live vector vaccines elicit potent immune responses against a foreign antigen in neonatal mice born to naive and immune mothers. Infect Immun. 2004;72(8):4637–46. https://doi.org/10.1128/IAI.72.8.4637-4646.2004. PMID: 15271924; PMCID: PMC470595.
60. Osman R, Malmuthuge N, Gonzalez-Cano P, Griebel P. Development and function of the Mucosal immune system in the upper respiratory tract of neonatal calves. Annu Rev Anim Biosci. 2018;6:141–55. https://doi.org/10.1146/annurev-animal-030117-014611. Epub 2017 Nov 6. PMID: 29106820.
61. Basha S, Surendran N, Pichichero M. Immune responses in neonates. Expert Rev Clin Immunol. 2014;10(9):1171–84. https://doi.org/10.1586/1744666X.2014.942288. Epub 2014 Aug 4. PMID: 25088080; PMCID: PMC4407563.
62. Bahroz A, Saleh M. Immunity Development in newborn calves: a review. ProEnvironment. 2022;15(50):187–96.
63. Torow N, Marsland BJ, Hornef MW, Gollwitzer ES. Neonatal mucosal immunology. Mucosal Immunol. 2017;10(1):5–17. https://doi.org/10.1038/mi.2016.81. Epub 2016 Sep 21. PMID: 27649929.
64. Oherle K, Acker E, Bonfield M, Wang T, Gray J, Lang I, Bridges J, Lewkowich I, Xu Y, Ahlfeld S, Zacharias W, Alenghat T, Deshmukh H. Insulin-like growth factor 1 supports a pulmonary niche that promotes type 3 innate lymphoid cell development in newborn lungs. Immunity. 2020;52(2):275–294.e9. https://doi.org/10.1016/j.immuni.2020.01.005. Erratum in: Immunity. 2020;52(4):716-718. doi: 10.1016/j.immuni.2020.03.018. PMID: 32075728; PMCID: PMC7382307.
65. Cardoso CL, King A, Chapwanya A, Esposito G. Ante-Natal and Post-Natal influences on neonatal immunity, growth and puberty of calves-a review. Animals Basel. 2021;11(5):1212. https://doi.org/10.3390/ani11051212. PMID: 33922339; PMCID: PMC8144962.

66. Cangiano LR, Villot C, Guan LL, Ipharraguerre IR, Steele MA. Graduate Student Literature Review: developmental adaptations of immune function in calves and the influence of the intestinal microbiota in health and disease. J Dairy Sci. 2024;107(4):2543–55.
67. Amin N, Seifert J. Dynamic progression of the calf's microbiome and its influence on host health. Comput Struct Biotechnol J. 2021;19:989–1001. https://doi.org/10.1016/j.csbj.2021.01.035. PMID: 33613865; PMCID: PMC7868804.
68. Chase CC, Hurley DJ, Reber AJ. Neonatal immune development in the calf and its impact on vaccine response. Vet Clin North Am Food Anim Pract. 2008;24(1):87–104. https://doi.org/10.1016/j.cvfa.2007.11.001. PMID: 18299033; PMCID: PMC7127081.
69. Mebus CA, White RG, Stair EL, Rhodes MB, Twiehaus MJ. Neonatal calf diarrhea: results of a field trial using a reo-like virus vaccine. Vet Med Small Anim Clin. 1972;67:173–4.
70. Zygraich N, Lobmann M, Vascoboinic E, Berge e, Huygelen C. In vivo and in vitro properties of a temperature sensitive mutant of infectious bovine Rhinotracheitis virus. Res Vet Sci. 1974;16(3):328–35. https://doi.org/10.1016/S0034-5288(18)33731-7. ISSN 0034-5288.
71. Wilson HL, Gerdts V, Babiuk LA. Mucosal vaccine development for veterinary and aquatic diseases. Mucosal Vaccines. 2020:811–829. https://doi.org/10.1016/B978-0-12-811924-2.00048-1. Epub 40. 2019 Oct 25. PMCID: PMC7149622.
72. Shewen PE, Carrasco-Medina L, BA MB, Hodgins DC. Challenges in mucosal vaccination of cattle. Vet Immunol Immunopathol. 2009;128(1–3):192–8. https://doi.org/10.1016/j.vetimm.2008.10.297. Epub 2008 Oct 17. PMID: 19046777; PMCID: PMC7127216.
73. Hodgins DC, Chattha K, Vlasova A, Parreño V, Corbeil LB, Renukaradhya GJ, Saif LJ. Mucosal veterinary vaccines: comparative vaccinology. In: Mucosal Immunol; 2015. p. 1337–61. https://doi.org/10.1016/B978-0-12-415847-4.00068-9. Epub 2015 Mar 13. PMCID: PMC7149859.
74. Lavelle EC, Ward RW. Mucosal vaccines – fortifying the frontiers. Nat Rev Immunol. 2022;22(4):236–50. https://doi.org/10.1038/s41577-021-00583-2. Epub 2021 Jul 26. Erratum in: Nat Rev Immunol. 2022;22(4):266. 10.1038/s41577-021-00599-8. PMID: 34312520; PMCID: PMC8312369.
75. Loehr BI, Willson P, Babiuk LA, van Drunen Little-van den Hurk S. Gene gun-mediated DNA immunization primes development of mucosal immunity against bovine herpesvirus-1 in cattle. J Virol. 2000;74:6077–86. https://doi.org/10.1128/jvi.74.13.6077-6086.2000.
76. Loehr BI, Rankin R, Pontarollo R, King T, Willson P, Babiuk LA, van Drunen Little-van den Hurk S. Suppository-mediated DNA immunization induces mucosal immunity against bovine herpesvirus-1 in cattle. Virology. 2001;289:327–33. https://doi.org/10.1006/viro.2001.1143.
77. Kit S, Kit M, McConnell S. Intramuscular and intravaginal vaccination of pregnant cows with thymidine kinase-negative, temperature-resistant infectious bovine rhinotracheitis virus (bovine herpes virus 1). Vaccine. 1986;4(1):55–61.
78. Cortese VS, Walz PH, Scruggs D, Short TH. Determination of protection provided by two modified live bovine herpesvirus-1 vaccines against bovine herpesvirus-1 conjunctivitis in calves. Bovine Pract. 2023;57(1):21–34.
79. Cravens RL, Bechtol DD. Clinical response of feeder calves under direct IBR and BVD virus challenge: a comparison of two Vaccines and negative control. Bovine Pract. 1991;26:154–8.

Neonatal Immunology

7

Abstract

As more is understood about the development of the calf's immune system, new opportunities for improving health and performance have been discovered. Influences on the developing and newborn calf impact their ability to mount an effective immune response and have long-term ramifications on the function of other body systems. As a result, understanding this critical period in a calf's life is vital to delivering effective bovine veterinary care that supports cattle operations and production goals.

Keywords

Neonatal immunology · Calf · Immune system development · Fetal development · Colostrum

Key Concepts

- While much of the immune system development occurs in utero, maturation of the immune system continues until sexual maturity is reached.
- The bovine fetus becomes immunocompetent during gestation to a variety of infections.
- At birth, the systemic immune system of the calf is well developed but immature. The local immune system is still developing.

J. Ellis, V. Cortese, *Practical Bovine Immunology*,
https://doi.org/10.1007/978-3-032-15031-8_7

How Does the Bovine Immune System Develop?

The immune system of all species of mammals begins development early in gestation. Thymic growth begins at 25 days of gestation in the calf [1, 2]. As the fetus grows, the immune system goes through many changes as cells appear and become specialized. In multiple species, stem cells that initially infiltrate the thymus primarily arise from the intra-embryonic aorta-gonad-mesonephros region. While this region has not been specifically implicated in the bovine fetus, it is generally accepted that hematopoietic stem cells sequentially seed various organs: first, the fetal liver, then the thymus and the spleen, and finally, the bone marrow [3]. These cells are the precursors of lymphoid and myeloid cell lineages. The lymphoid cell lineage develops into the natural killer cells and B and T lymphocytes, while the myeloid cell lineage gives rise to granulocytes, including neutrophils, eosinophils, and basophils.

During gestation, the *thymus* is the primary organ for the development and differentiation of thymocytes into specific lineages of *T lymphocytes*, each with specific "*CD*" (cluster of differentiation; Chap. 4) markers. This begins as early as day 42 of gestation in the bovine fetus [4]. *B cells*, by contrast, in most mammals, develop and differentiate in the fetal bone marrow. However, in cattle, sheep, and other ungulates, the major site for these processes is the *ileal Peyer's patches* [5, 6] add reference 6 after 5, which are, therefore, considered to be the primary lymphoid organ for B cells in those species.

The majority of circulating fetal lymphocytes are T cells, but other leukocytes are also developing and expanding in the bovine fetus. Eventually, immunocompetent T and B lymphocytes reach secondary lymphoid tissues. Lymph nodes are visible by day 60, while Peyer's patches are not seen until day 175 [4]. Here, and in other secondary lymphoid organs, immune responses to specific antigens of microbes occur in the bovine fetus and the newborn calf. In the fetal calf, this immune responsiveness has been demonstrated with a wide variety of infections [7–14] at various times of fetal life (Table 7.1). It should be noted that very few of these specific days are indicative of when the fetus is actually "first" able to respond, as there is some individual variability, and the studies were not performed at different fetal ages to determine at what age the fetal immune response was initially able to occur.

The practical implication of this early ability to respond is that for intrauterine infections, notably bovine viral diarrhea virus (BVDV), precolostral titers from the neonate can be used for diagnostic determination of fetal exposures, once the virus has come and gone by the time of birth, and would often be undetectable by other means. As well, the ability to respond may also give the fetus some ability to decrease the severity of the disease if an intrauterine infection occurs.

Table 7.1 Examples of agents and approximate ages at which immune reactivity in the bovine fetus was found [4, 14]

Age (days in gestation)	Agents
Day 73	Rotavirus
Day 76	Cache Valley virus -
Day 95	Bovine viral diarrhea virus
Day 120	Bovine parainfluenza virus -3
Day 122	Bluetongue virus
Day 203	*Escherichia coli*

In the thymus, undeveloped T lymphocytes proliferate and mature into antigen-specific T cells. An individual T cell can only recognize a single epitope comprising either self or non-self-antigens via T cell receptors (Chap. 4). During maturation in the thymus, clones of T lymphocytes differentiate into either CD4-expressing T helper lymphocytes or CD8-expressing cytotoxic lymphocytes. Most of the developing T lymphocytes in the thymus die by *apoptosis* (programmed cell death) (>95%) via positive and negative selective processes. During maturation, T lymphocytes move into deeper parts of the cortex, where the expression of CD4 or CD8 is initiated [3].

Precursor B lymphocytes initially replicate and mature to form cells individually committed to recognize only one epitope on either "self" or "non-self" antigens through their B cell receptors (BCRs; Chap. 3). The BCRs are immunoglobulins of the IgM type that are membrane-bound antibodies. B lymphocytes are also chosen through positive and negative selection processes. Mature, naïve B lymphocytes will leave the bovine ileal Peyer's patch, circulate in the blood and lymph, and colonize secondary lymphatic tissues [3–5; Chap. 3].

What Factors Contribute to the Immaturity of Immune Responses in the Calf?

At the time of birth, a neonate's systemic immune system is fully developed, albeit at an immature level. In contrast, the local immune system is still undergoing development (Chap. 6). Susceptibility of the newborn to pathogens is not due to any inherent inability to mount an immune response, but is because their immune system is unprimed and immature [7, 15]. This immaturity affects the efficiency of both innate and adaptive responses.

Although there are relatively higher numbers of phagocytic cells, neutrophils, and macrophages in the neonate, the function of these cells is decreased, especially around birth, because of high steroid levels. These deficiencies can be found up to 4 months of age [15, 16]. Complement components are from 12% to 60% of adult levels at birth, resulting in poor opsonic activity. Complement will not reach adult levels in calves until they are 6 months of age. Despite this immaturity in innate immune responses, calves are relatively more dependent on them because of the immaturity of their adaptive immune system early in life [14].

There is also a slow maturation of the adaptive immune system in mammals. As cattle approach sexual maturity, the immune system also matures. In cattle, most of the immune system is considered "mature" by 5–8 months of age. For example, T cells (CD4+, CD8+, and TCRγδ+) do not reach peak levels until the animal is 8 months of age [16]. Compared to the much more-studied immune systems of mice and humans, a different feature of the bovine (as well as other ruminants and pigs) immune system is the preponderance of *γδ T cells* in the neonate and young calf; as much as 60% of circulating T cells in the young calf are γδ T cells [16, 17; Chap. 5]. What these cells are actually doing immunologically is not completely resolved; in many ways, they act more like an innate effector cell than CD4+ and CD8+ T cells [17]. Nevertheless, simply decreasing the relative proportions of "conventional," more antigen-specific αβ T cells (CD4+ and CD8+) could affect the state of "maturity" of the adaptive immune response in the neonate. In addition, calves, like human infants, are said to have a "*T-helper 2 (Th2) bias*" in their adaptive responses [18, 19]. A *Th2 bias* refers to a skewing of the immune response toward the *Th2 pathway*, which is associated with antibody production and responses to extracellular pathogens such as bacteria and parasites, as well as with the production of interleukin (IL)-4, IL-5, IL-10, and IL-13 [18, 19; Chap. 4]. This bias can make them more susceptible to *intracellular pathogens* such as viruses and certain bacteria, which require a *Th1-type response* (involving cell-mediated immunity) for effective clearance. The Th2 dominance may also influence how calves respond to vaccines and infections, potentially leading to *suboptimal protection* if the immune system does not adequately shift toward a balanced or Th1-dominant response as they mature.

All of this does not mean that a young calf cannot respond to antigens, notably in vaccines [20, 21]. Young calves have been shown to develop disease-sparing responses to vaccination, but these responses will generally be weaker, slower to develop, easier to overcome, and can be variably inhibited by maternal antibodies [22, 23]. These limitations should be conveyed to clients. Actual regression of the thymus begins around puberty, and the extent and speed at which it regresses will vary by husbandry practices and genetics. By the time of the first heat cycle, the thymus's function as a lymphoid organ is almost completely gone. The ileal Peyer's patch also involutes along a similar timeline, and B lymphocytes take up residence in the bone marrow and secondary lymphoid tissues and organs, including other Peyer's patches found in the intestines of the adult animal [5]. This immaturity of immune responses may lead to moderation of disease rather than complete prevention. Since the placenta is of the epitheliochorial type in food animal species (cattle, pigs, and sheep), there is no transplacental transfer of antibodies or white blood cells. Therefore, no discussion on bovine neonatal immunology is complete without a discussion on an important component of the newborn calf's defense mechanism, colostrum.

What Are the Immunologically Important Components of Colostrum?

Colostrum is the most important example of natural, passive immunity in cattle. Defined as the "first" secretions from the mammary gland present after birth, colostrum has many known and unknown properties and components. The information on both the short- and long-term impacts of colostrum in calves continues to grow, and there is a large body of research that has been published on colostrum in calves. Not only does good passive transfer impact morbidity and mortality in the young calf [24–27], but it also has a positive impact on long-term health and production [27–29]. The primary antibody and most important component of colostrum in most domestic species is immunoglobulin isotype G; in ruminants, subclass immunoglobulin G1 (IgG1) predominates [30]. Additional soluble components of the immune system, such as interferon and other cytokines, lactoferrin, and antimicrobial peptides, are also transferred via colostrum [30, 31]. More recently, microRNAs that modulate the expression of genes coding for factors involved in immune function and intestinal development have been measured in bovine colostrum [31].

In addition to soluble factors, there are also high numbers of white blood cells in the colostrum of cattle and other species. Bovine colostrum has approximately 10^6 leukocytes/mL, and, depending on the stage of lactation, macrophages and neutrophils comprise the majority of colostral white blood cells, followed by lymphocytes [32, 33]. T lymphocytes represent a higher proportion of lymphocytes than B lymphocytes, at 16% and 10.7% of the total white blood cells, respectively [32, 33]. The majority of lymphocytes are of the memory phenotype [32, 33]. The colostral substrate enhances the ability of lymphocytes to cross the intestinal barrier and enter the systemic circulation in the newborn calf [32, 33] and also affects the trafficking patterns of the absorbed lymphocytes. But, essentially, absorption of colostral leukocytes, through and between intestinal epithelial cells, is a non-specific process [33].

Numerous laboratory studies have demonstrated that colostral leukocytes can be involved in a variety of immunological phenomena in the neonate, including: transfer of delayed type hypersensitivity, lymphocyte blastogenic responses to mitogens, antigen-specific responses to microbial and vaccinal antigens, local bactericidal and phagocytic activity in the digestive tract, and enhanced passive transfer of immunoglobulins [31–33].

The reason colostral leukocytes are able to interact immunologically with various cells in the calf is that mother and offspring are *semi-allogeneic* (same species, different individual), meaning that they share some of the same molecules that are essential to antigen presentation—the majority histocompatibility complex (MHC) molecules [33; Chap. 4. This means that calf lymphocytes can respond to antigens presented by maternal antigen-presenting cells and vice versa. As well, maternal T lymphocytes can respond to antigens "presented" on the MHC molecules expressed on microbe-infected cells in the calf, or by other, "professional" antigen-presenting cells [e.g., dendritic cells;]. Importantly, these interactions can only occur between calves and maternal cells that share the same MHC molecules, but not between leukocytes from other (unrelated) cows, or in pooled raw colostrum, a common first feeding source. This is because most of the leukocytes in pooled colostrum would be (completely) *allogeneic*, sharing few if any MHC molecules. No microbial antigen-specific interactions can occur between MHC-mismatched cells; that is one of the central dogmas of immunology [33]. This *MHC restriction* has been demonstrated for both CD8+ and CD4+ T cells in cattle as well [34, 35], even though, primarily due to inbreeding, the bovine MHC is less *polymorphic* (variable) than more outbred species, notably humans [36, 37].

So, why do colostral leukocytes "disappear" from the calf in a few weeks, when cells like macrophages and memory T cells would generally be much longer lived, even for years? (Chap. 4) Although it has not been completely investigated in cattle, the best explanation can be found in the much-studied field of transplantation biology [38, 39]. In many ways, maternal colostral leukocytes behave like an *allograft or semi-allograft*, a "transplant" between two individuals of the same species that are not identical twins. Even though there is some degree of immunological tolerance in neonates [40], much like the fate of a maternal kidney or bone marrow transplant, maternal colostral leukocytes are probably "*rejected*" by the calf, in a matter of weeks after birth, because they are semi-allogenic (to the calf) and *do not share all* of the same MHC molecules. This rejection process would be even more vigorous in the case of MHC-mismatched leukocytes in pooled raw (fully allogeneic) colostrum. Imagine a maternal T cell that has trafficked to a lymph node in a calf. It can be presented with an antigen by the calf's dendritic (antigen-presenting) cells, but can also be attacked by the calf's *allo-specific T cells*, which are highly prevalent in T cell populations of all species [39–41]. This "attack" happens because the colostral T cell will be recognized as "foreign" (different MHC molecules). Conversely, other colostral T cells with allo-specificities can interact with the calf's cells in *graft-versus-host* reactions. Overall, rejection, and allo-specific reactions in general are robust immunological processes, involving a variety of cells and cytokines. An important "bystander" effect of this process is, undoubtedly, activation of the calf's immune system [38, 39]. Indeed, many of the effects of colostral leukocytes, including their "disappearance" by 3–5 weeks of age, and their "activational" and "educational" effects on the calf's immune system, are probably best explained by these proinflammatory allogenic interactions [38, 39, 42].

Due to all the variabilities in neonatal disease and the myriad of colostral components that may be involved in formulating neonatal immune responses, there are few studies that demonstrate the overall effect of the ingestion of viable colostral leukocytes on calf health. Colostral leukocytes are not necessary to avert morbidity and mortality in conventionally reared calves. The best practical proof of that is the common practice of raising healthy calves with frozen or refrigerated pooled colostrum, but, almost certainly, colostral leukocytes aid in rearing the young calf. Furthermore, maternal cells are not necessary to develop disease-sparing responses to vaccines, as documented in numerous vaccine efficacy studies, mostly using calves that are either colostrum negative or have not received viable colostral leukocytes or antigen-specific antibodies.

The presence or absence of viable colostral leukocytes is mostly an issue in dairies where colostrum management is an important component of the calf program. Collection, pooling, inventory control, and storage to increase shelf-life, as well as pooling and processing by freezing, pasteurization, or spray drying, or adding preservatives, are all utilized on dairies. Some of these "kill" cells, as well as bacteria and viruses. This means that colostral leukocytes are mainly a management issue in dairy cattle, as most beef calves will receive at least some colostrum directly from the dam. In one large randomized study involving over 1000 dairy calves that received pooled colostrum with viable colostral leukocytes, or pooled pasteurized colostrum in which the leukocytes were significantly reduced, it was the calves that received the pasteurized colostrum that had reduced morbidity and better health outcomes [43, 44]. These results indicate that microbial contamination, and the reduction thereof by processing, is a more important factor in calf health than the availability of all of colostral leukocytes in "managed" colostrum; however, it should be noted that pasteurization does not destroy all colostral leukocytes [44].

How Is Colostrum Absorbed in the Newborn Calf?

When calves are born, the epithelial cells that line the digestive tract allow absorption of colostral proteins via pinocytosis. As soon as the digestive tract is stimulated by the ingestion of any material, this population of cells begins to change to those that no longer permit absorption. By 6 h after birth, only about 50% of the absorptive capacity remains, by 8 h 33%, and by 24 h, no absorption is typically seen [30]. Colostrum transfer is a function of the quality and quantity of the colostrum as well as the timing of colostral administration. The first colostral feeding or nursing should be within the first 2 hours of life [30, 45–48]. In the Holstein breed, the first feeding should be a minimum of 3 quarts (3 L) and preferably 4 quarts of high-quality, clean colostrum [30, 45–48]. Feeding colostrum high in red blood cells should be avoided as it may exacerbate any diarrhea caused by Gram-negative bacteria [30]. Additionally, *stress, cold exposure, or dystocia* can impair a calf's ability to stand and nurse, delaying colostrum intake and reducing absorption. In spite of all of the information regarding the importance of colostrum administration to the calf, some degree of failure of passive transfer is common even in beef calves [30, 45–48].

Many colostrum replacements and supplements, including whole colostrum, fractionated colostrum, and blood-derived products, are available, usually for oral administration. There is significant variability in the IgG concentration in colostral supplements/replacers [30, 49], and they do not contain viable colostral leukocytes. A good indicator of reasonable expectations for efficacy of the various products is documentation of the functional IgG1 concentration. Although mixed results have been observed pertaining to the efficacy of these products [30, 50, 51] in colostrum-deprived calves or calves with poor passive transfer, they can have a significant value in decreasing the mortality and/or severity of the disease [30, 50, 51]. Colostrum-based products can also be given *post-day 1* to reduce perinatal morbidity and mortality and promote growth. In that case, since the gut would be closed to passive absorption of proteins, the disease-sparing effects would be due to local effects of antibodies and antimicrobial proteins (lactoferrin) and the anabolic effects of colostral fat and growth factors [52].

There are several different methods to assess passive transfer /IgG concentrations in calves from day 1 to 7 of age. While radial immunodiffusion is the gold standard method and directly measures IgG concentration, serum total protein, an indirect measurement, is the most common method used today [30, 53, 54]. The current research indicates that serum total protein of at least 6.0 g/dL is a reasonable measure of adequate passive transfer [30, 55–59]. The best predictor of young calf health is a serum IgG concentration of 10 g/L [30]; however, it should be noted that the higher IgG concentration also correlates to higher levels of other components of colostrum as well.

Can Vaccinating the Cow Improve Colostral Antibody Levels?

It has long been thought that vaccines administered to a cow before calving will increase colostral antibodies against those specific antigens. This has been best demonstrated with vaccines against neonatal diarrhea pathogens that are administered to cows. These vaccines are designed to increase the colostral antibody concentration against specific organisms that cause diarrhea in calves, such as *E. coli*, rotavirus, *Clostridium perfringens,* and coronavirus [60–62]. For these vaccines, timing to provide an adequate immune response in cows and movement of antibodies into the colostrum is important.

However, little research has been done looking at other vaccines and their impact on colostral antibodies, and much of the available data are conflicting. While one study demonstrated that vaccinating cows with a modified live viral vaccine increased colostral antibodies [63], another study with inactivated viral vaccination of previously vaccinated cows did not show the same response [64]. Further complicating the matter are data demonstrating decreased colostral antibodies when cows were vaccinated with some antigens before calving [64]. A vaccine claiming to be used primarily to improve colostral transfer of antibodies should have evidence-based support in the form of well-designed field-based trials.

Why Is Stress Important in the Newborn Calf?

Stress impacts the calf's immune system as it does in older animals. There are several factors that can affect the immune system that are unique to the neonatal animal. The calving process has a dramatic impact on the newborn's systemic immune system due to corticosteroid release [3, 30]. This factor, along with others, dramatically decreases systemic immune responses for the first week of life. Vaccination immediately after birth may even have undesired effects, especially if there is poor passive transfer. Furthermore, other stresses should be avoided in the young calf to try and maintain immune system integrity in the immunologically frail newborn. Procedures such as castration, dehorning, weaning, and movement need to be considered as stresses that have the potential to decrease immune system function temporarily.

Conclusion

The neonatal immune system is a complex and interrelated system containing components from both the dam and the newborn. Although the system is capable of responding and inferring varying degrees of protection, it is this combination of passive and active immunity together that provides protection to the neonate. Research continues to provide information on methods for improving health during this critical period.

Your Case

History and Problem

500 cow/calf operation in Kansas. The commercial angus herd is split into two herds: a spring calving herd of approximately 300 cows and a fall calving herd of 200 cows. The herd is bull bred, utilizing approximately 20 bulls, which are rotated through both sets of cows. There is a 25% bull replacement rate per year. The fall herd is halfway through calving and experiencing scours in 20–25% of the calves. Initially, the diarrhea started at 10–14 days of age, but it is slowly moving into younger calves (current cases have an onset of 7 days). The majority of calves have been treated by the rancher; only five calves have required veterinary intervention with systemic fluids and supportive care, but three out of five calves died.

Pertinent Background Information

Cows are brought into two large pastures, close to the ranch house for calving. Heifers are kept in separate pastures from the cows until they are moved into the calving pastures with the cows. The majority of affected calves are from heifers. The herd is on an annual modified live bovine herpesvirus 1 (BHV-1), bovine parainfluenza virus-3 (BPIV-3), bovine respiratory syncytial virus (BRSV), and BVDV types 1 and 2 containing a five-*Leptospira* bacterin. Calves are vaccinated at approximately 60 days of age with a *Clostridial* eight-way bacterin-toxoid vaccine and an intranasal modified live BHV-1, BPIV-3, BRSV vaccine, and are moved onto the modified live vaccination program at preweaning and weaning.

Questions for You

1. How do you start to diagnose the underlying cause of the scours outbreak?
2. What follow-up testing do you do based on the initial results?
3. What are your recommendations to control this outbreak and prevent it next year?

Additional Readings

1. Hubbert WT, Stalheim OHV, Booth GD. Changes in organ weights and fluid volumes during growth of the bovine fetus. Growth. 1972;36:217–33.
2. Anderson EI. Pharyngeal derivatives in the calf. Anat Rec. 1922;24:25–37.
3. Vejlsted M. Chapter 13: Development of the immune system. In: Hyttel P, Sinowatz F, Vejlsted M, editors. Essentials of domestic animals embryology. Amsterdam: Saunders Elsevier; 2009. p. 208–15.
4. Schultz RD, Dunne HW, Heist CE. Ontogeny of the bovine immune response. Infect Immunol. 1973;7(6):981–91.
5. Yasuda M, Jenne CN, Kennedy LJ, Reynolds JD. The sheep and cattle Peyer's patch as a site of B-cell development. Vet Res. 2006;37:401–15.
6. Senogles DR, Muscoplat CC, Paul PS, Johnson DW. Ontogeny of circulating B lymphocytes in neonatal calves. Res Vet Sci. 1978;25:34–6.

7. Halliwell REW, Gorman NT. Neonatal immunology. In: Veterinary clinical immunology. Philadelphia: W.B. Saunders Co; 1989. p. 193–205.
8. Mullaney TP, Newman LE, Whitehair CK. Humoral immune response of the bovine fetus to in utero vaccination with attenuated bovine coronavirus. Am J Vet Res. 1988;49:156–9.
9. Torres MP, Ortega YR. Neospora caninum antibodies in commercial fetal bovine serum. Vet Parasitol. 2006;140(3–4):352–5.
10. Ellsworth MA, Fairbanks KK, Behan S, Jackson JA, Goodyear M, Oien NL, Meinert TR, Leyh RD. Fetal protection following exposure to calves persistently infected with bovine viral diarrhea virus type 2 sixteen months after primary vaccination of the dams. Vet Therapeut. 2006;7:295–304.
11. Conner GH, Richardson M, Carter GR, Wamukoya JP. Immune responses of the bovine fetus. J Dairy Sci. 1977;60(2):289–93. https://doi.org/10.3168/jds.S0022-0302(77)83867-8. PMID: 320237; PMCID: PMC7130515.
12. Kelling CL, Topliff CL. Bovine maternal, fetal and neonatal responses to bovine viral diarrhea virus infections. Biologicals. 2013;41(1):20–5. https://doi.org/10.1016/j.biologicals.2012.09.006. Epub 2012 Oct 17. PMID: 23084809.
13. Pinto GB, Hawkes P, Zábal O, Ulloa E, Lager IA, Weber EL, Schudel AA. Viral antibodies in bovine fetuses in Argentina. Res Vet Sci. 1993;55(3):385–8. https://doi.org/10.1016/0034-5288(93)90114-u. PMID: 8284507; PMCID: PMC7131699.
14. Tizard I. Immunity in the fetus and newborn. In: Veterinary immunology, an introduction. 10th ed. Philadelphia: W.B. Sanders Co.; 2018. p. 264–78.
15. Hawser MA, Knob MD, Roth JA. Variation of neutrophil function with age in calves. Am J Vet Res. 1986;47:152–3.
16. Hein WR. Ontogeny of T cells. In: Goddeeris BML, Morrison WI, editors. Cell mediated immunity in ruminants. CRC press; 1994. p. 19–36.
17. Baldwin CL, Damani-Yokota P, Yirsaw A, et al. Special features of γδ T cells in ruminants. Mol Immunol. 2021;124:161–9. https://doi.org/10.1016/j.molimm.2021.02.028.
18. Eder JM, Sacco RE. Ex vivo activated $CD4^{+}$ T cells from young calves exhibit Th2-biased effector function with distinct metabolic reprogramming compared to adult cows. Vet Immunol Immunopathol. 2022;248:110418. https://doi.org/10.1016/j.vetimm.2022.110418. Epub 2022 Apr 12. PMID: 35447485.
19. Debock I, Flamand V. Unbalanced neonatal CD4+ T cell immunity. Front Immunol. 2014;2014:5. https://doi.org/10.3389/fimmu.2014.00393.
20. Cortese VS, West KH, Hassard LE, Carman S, Ellis JA. Clinical and immunologic responses of vaccinated and unvaccinated calves to infection with a virulent type-II isolate of bovine viral diarrhea virus. J Am Vet Med Assoc. 1998;213(9):1312–9.
21. West KH, Petrie L, Konoby C, et al. The efficacy of modified-live bovine respiratory syncytial virus vaccines in experimentally infected calves. Vaccine. 1999;18:907–19. https://doi.org/10.1016/S0264-410X(99)00324-2.
22. Ellis J, West K, Cortese V, Konoby C, Weigel D. Effect of maternal antibodies on induction and persistence of vaccine-induced immune responses against bovine viral diarrhea virus type II in young calves. JAVMA. 2001;219:351–6.
23. Ellis J, Gow S, Bolton M, Burdett W, Nordstrom S. Inhibition of priming for bovine respiratory syncytial virus-specific protective immune responses following parenteral vaccination of passively immune calves. Can Vet J. 2014;55(12):1180–5. PMID: 25477547; PMCID: PMC4231808.
24. Boland W, Cortese VS, Steffen D. Interactions between vaccination, failure of passive transfer, and diarrhea in beef calves. Agric Pract. 1995;16:25–8.
25. Robison AD, Stott GH, DeNise SK. Effects of passive immunity on growth and survival in the dairy heifer. J Dairy Sci. 1988;71:1283–7.
26. Cortese VS, Kirkpatrick MA, Short TH, Voortman B. Effect of serum total protein concentration on early-life health and growth of dairy calves. J Am Vet Med Assoc. 2020;257(1):80–8.
27. Faber SN, Pas, Faber NE, Ax RL. Case study: effects of colostrum ingestion on lactational performance. Prof Anim Sci. 2005;21:420–5.

28. Wittum TE, Perino LJ. Passive immune status at postpartum hour 24 and long-term health and performance of calves. Am J Vet Res. 1995;56:1149–54.
29. Dewell RD, Hungerford LL, Keen JE, Laegreid WW, Griffin DD, Rupp GP, Grotelueschen DM. Association of neonatal serum immunoglobulin G1 concentration with health and performance in beef calves. J Am Vet Med Assoc. 2006;228:914–21.
30. Godden SM, Lombard JE, Woolums AR. Colostrum management for dairy calves. Vet Clin Food Anim 2019; 35: 19–39. Vet Clin North Am Food Anim Pract. 2019;35:535–56. https://doi.org/10.1016/j.cvfa.2019.07.005.
31. Rostoll-Cangiano L, Cid de la Paz M, Pierre JF. Beyond immunoglobulin G: dissecting the role of colostrum in programming early immune function in calves. JDS Commun. 2025;6:474–8.
32. Gonzalez DD, Dus Santos MJ. Bovine colostral cells—the often forgotten component of colostrum. J Am Vet Med Assoc. 2017;250:998–1005.
33. Ellis J. Passive transfer of colostral leukocytes: a benefit/risk analysis. Can Vet J. 2021;62:233–9.
34. Graham SP, Pellé R, Yamage M, Mwangi DM, et al. Characterization of the fine specificity of bovine CD8 T-cell responses to defined antigens from the protozoan parasite Theileria parva. Infect Immun. 2008;76(2):685–94. https://doi.org/10.1128/IAI.01244-07. Epub 2007 Dec 10. PMID: 18070892; PMCID: PMC2223472.
35. Mitoma S, Carr BV, Harvey Y. The detection of long- lasting memory foot-and- mouth disease(FMD) virus serotype O-specific CD4+ T cells from FMD-vaccinated cattle by bovine major histocompatibility complex class II tetramer. Immunology. 2021;164:266–78.
36. Ellis SA, Morrison WI, MacHugh ND, Birch J, Burrells A, Stear MJ. Serological and molecular diversity in the cattle MHC class I region. Immunogenetics. 2005;57(8):601–6. https://doi.org/10.1007/s00251-005-0027-8. Epub 2005 Sep 29. PMID: 16086171.
37. Ellis SA, Codner G. The impact of MHC diversity on cattle T cell responses. Vet Immunol Immunopathol. 2012;148:74–7. https://doi.org/10.1016/j.vetimm.2011.03.009.
38. Moreau A, Varey E, Anegon I, Cuturi MC. Effector mechanisms of rejection. Cold Spring Harb Perspect Med. 2013;3:a015461. https://doi.org/10.1101/cshperspect.a015461. PMC 3808773. PMID 24186491.
39. Marino J, Paster J, Benichou G. Allorecognition by T lymphocytes and allograft rejection. Front Immunol. 2016;7:582. https://doi.org/10.3389/fimmu.2016.00582. PMID: 28018349; PMCID: PMC5155009.
40. Robinson KA, Orent W, Madsen JC, Benichou G. Maintaining T cell tolerance of alloantigens: lessons from animal studies. Am J Transplant. 2018;18(8):1843–56. https://doi.org/10.1111/ajt.14984. PMID: 29939471; PMCID: PMC6352985.
41. Teale AJ, Morrison WI, Goddeeris BM, Groocock CM, Stagg DA, Spooner RL. Bovine alloreactive cytotoxic cells generated in vitro: target specificity in relation to BoLA phenotype. Immunology. 1985;55(2):355–62. PMID: 2409001; PMCID: PMC1453610.
42. Reber AJ, Hippen AR, Hurley DJ. Effects of the ingestion of whole colostrum or cell-free colostrum on the capacity of leukocytes in newborn calves to stimulate or respond in one-way mixed leukocyte cultures. Am J Vet Res. 2005;66(11):1854–60. https://doi.org/10.2460/ajvr.2005.66.1854.
43. Godden SM, Smolenski DJ, Donahue M, Oakes BR, Wells S, Sreevatsan S, Stabel J, Fetrow J. Heat-treated colostrum and reduced morbidity in preweaned dairy calves: results of a randomized trial and examination of mechanisms of effectiveness. J Dairy Sci. 2012;95:4029–40.
44. Mann S, Curone G, Chandler TL, Moroni P, Cha J, Bhawal R, Zhang S. Heat treatment of bovine colostrum: I. Effects on bacterial and somatic cell counts, immunoglobulin, insulin, and IGF-I concentrations, as well as the colostrum proteome. J Dairy Sci. 2020;103(10):9368–83. ISSN/ISBN: 1525-3198 PMID: 32828510.
45. Urie NJ, Lombard JE, Shivley CB, Kopral CA, Adams AE, Earleywine TJ, Olson JD, Garry FB. Preweaned heifer management on US dairy operations: part I. Descriptive characteristics of preweaned heifer raising practices. J Dairy Sci. 2018;101:9168–84.
46. Todd CG, McGee M, Tiernan K, Crosson P, O'Riordan E, McClure J, Lorenz I, Earley B. An observational study on passive immunity in Irish suckler beef and dairy calves: tests for failure of passive transfer of immunity and associations with health and performance. Prev Vet Med. 2018;159:182–95. https://doi.org/10.1016/j.prevetmed.2018.07.014. ISSN 0167-5877.

47. McGee M, Earley B. Review: passive immunity in beef-suckler calves. Animal. 2019;13(4):810–25.
48. Courtney AK, Epperson WB, Wittig TA, Pruitt RJ. Defining Failure of Passive Transfer in South Dakota Beef Calves. South Dakota Beef Report, 2000. Paper 16. http://openprairie.sdstate.edu/sd_beefreport_2000/16
49. Haines DM, Chelack BJ, Naylor JM. Immunoglobulin concentrations in commercially available colostrum supplements for calves. Can Vet J. 1990;31:36–7.
50. Grigaleviciute R, Planciuniene R, Prikockyte I, Radzeviciute-Valciuke E, Baleviciute A, Zelvys A, Zinkeviciene A, Zigmantaite V, Kucinskas A, Matusevicius P, Kavaliauskas P. The influence of feeding with colostrum and colostrum replacer on major blood biomarkers and growth performance in dairy calves. Vet Sci. 2023;10(2):128. https://doi.org/10.3390/vetsci10020128. PMID: 36851432; PMCID: PMC9965887.
51. Priestley D, Bittar JH, Ibarbia L, Risco CA, Galvão KN. Effect of feeding maternal colostrum or plasma-derived or colostrum-derived colostrum replacer on passive transfer of immunity, health, and performance of preweaning heifer calves. J Dairy Sci. 2013;96(5):3247–56. https://doi.org/10.3168/jds.2012-6339. Epub 2013 Mar 15
52. McCarthy HR, Cantor MC, Lopez AJ, et al. Effects of supplementing colostrum beyond the first day of life on growth and health parameters of preweaning Holstein heifers. J Dairy Sci. 2024;107:3280–91. https://doi.org/10.3168/jds.2023-23649.
53. de Souza RS, Dos Santos LBC, Melo IO, Cerqueira DM, Dumas JV, Leme FOP, Moreira TF, Meneses RM, de Carvalho AU, Facury-Filho EJ. Current diagnostic methods for assessing transfer of passive immunity in calves and possible improvements: a literature review. Animals (Basel). 2021;11(10):2963. https://doi.org/10.3390/ani11102963. PMID: 34679982; PMCID: PMC8532593.
54. Atkinson DJ, von Keyserlingk MAG, Weary DM. Benchmarking passive transfer of immunity and growth in dairy calves. J Dairy Sci. 2017;100(5):3773–82. https://doi.org/10.3168/jds.2016-11800. ISSN 0022-0302.
55. Donovan GA, Dohoo IR, Montgomery DM, Bennett FL. Associations between passive immunity and morbidity and mortality in dairy heifers in Florida, USA. Prevent Vet Med. 1998;34:31–46.
56. Van Amburgh ME, Soberon F, Lopez DJ, Karszes J, Everett RW. Early life nutrition and management impacts long-term productivity of calves. In: 50th Florida dairy production conference, Gainesville, Fl; 2014. p. 35–48.
57. McCarthy HR, Cantor MC, Lopez AJ, et al. Effects of supplementing colostrum beyond the first day of life on growth and health parameters of preweaning Holstein heifers. J Dairy Sci. 2024;107(5):3280–91. https://doi.org/10.3168/jds.2023-23649.
58. Soberon F, Van Amburgh ME. Effects of colostrum intake and pre-weaning nutrient intake on post-weaning feed efficiency and voluntary feed intake. J Dairy Sci. 2011;94(E suppl. 1):69. (abstr.)
59. Saif LJ, Smith KL, Landmeier BJ, Bohl EH, Theil KW, Todhunter DA. Immune response of pregnant cows to bovine rotavirus immunization. Am J Vet Res. 1984;45(1):49–58.
60. Saif LJ, Redmen DR, Smith KL, Thiel KW. Passive immunity to bovine rotavirus in newborn calves fed colstrum supplements from immunized or nonimmunized cows. Infect Immun. 1983;41:1118–31.
61. Murakami T, Hirano N, Inoue A, Chitose K, Tsuchiya K, Ono K, Naito Y. Tranfer of antibodies against viruses of calf diarrhea from cows to their offspring via colostrum. Jpn J Vet Sci. 1985;47:507–10.
62. Osterstock JB, Callan RJ, Van Metre DC. Evaluation of dry cow vaccination with a killed viral vaccine on post-colostral antibody titers in calves. Proc Am Assoc Bov Pract. 2003;36:163–4.
63. Brenner J, Samina I, Machanai B, Friedman S, Effron Y. Impact of vaccination of pregnant cows on colostral IgG levels and on term of pregnancy. Field observations. Israel J Vet Med. 1997;52(2–3):56–9.
64. Bryan LA, Fenton RA, Misra V, Haines DM. Fatal, generalized bovine herpesvirus type-1 infection associated with a modified-live infectious bovine rhinotracheitis/parainfluenza-3 vaccine administered to neonatal calves. Can Vet J. 1994;35(4):223–8.

Nutrition and Immunity in Cattle

8

Abstract

The impact that nutrition has on a properly functioning immune system is multiplied in cattle due to production systems that could cause nutritional deficiencies or toxicities in large groups of cattle, rather than in an individual animal. Since nutrition has such a big influence on proper immune system function, understanding the impact various nutrients can have on the immune system is important for understanding the potential for immune system failure in production animals. The nutritional status of cattle requires appropriate feed intake and proper supplements matched to the animal's production use, physiological condition, overall health, and reproductive status, and balanced with the feed, all of which can influence the function of the immune system. Therefore, bovine veterinary practitioners must consider energy balance, protein, trace minerals, and vitamin status that may affect the animal's immune response.

Keywords

Nutrition and immunology · Vitamins · Micro-minerals · Macro-minerals · Protein · Energy · Microbiota · Rumen health

Key Concepts

- The immune system is dependent on proper nutrition to function correctly.
- Energy and protein deficiencies can cause immune system failure.
- Other nutrient deficiencies (macro- and micro-minerals and vitamins) can cause decreased immune responses by affecting specific portions of the immune system.

J. Ellis, V. Cortese, *Practical Bovine Immunology*,
https://doi.org/10.1007/978-3-032-15031-8_8

Why Are We Discussing Nutrition in an Immunology Textbook?

Nothing has a bigger impact on the immune system in production animals than proper nutrition (Table 8.1). *Nutritional imbalances* can not only cause immune dysfunction but also exacerbate disease, increase susceptibility to infections, or increase the likelihood of adverse reactions. Whether it is deficiencies or toxicities, imbalances in both micro- and macro-minerals, essential nutrients, and vitamins can adversely impact the immune system [1]. The most consistent abnormalities are seen in cell-mediated immunity, complement system, phagocyte function, cytokine production, mucosal secretory antibody response, and antibody affinity [2].

What Major Nutrients Are Important for Proper Immune System Function?

Water is the most important nutrient for cattle. A water deficiency will result in death far more quickly than a deficiency of any other nutrient. Restricting water intake can decrease the animal's resiliency to environmental stressors, decrease feed intake, and directly and indirectly affect immune function. Energy and protein are required for every single process within the body, including the immune system. Energy serves as fuel for the synthesis and function of immune cells, whereas protein regulates and serves as a structural component for cells and antibodies. Many immune system components, such as cytokines (that control the growth and activity of immune cells) and antibodies, are vital proteins that are necessary for optimal immune function.

Protein-energy malnutrition (PEM) is most often seen in calves, particularly dairy calves [3], on limited nutrient intakes or cattle undergoing severe cold weather stress. Energy requirements of cattle depend on age, sex, body size, physiological state, and environment. PEM can lead to increased frequency and severity of infections [2]. Proper activation and maintenance of the immune response requires adequate energy and protein. During acute infection, if an animal is energy-deficient, it

Table 8.1 Impact of various nutrients on immune system function

		Adaptive immune system	
Nutrient	Innate immune system	T cells	B cells
Protein	X	X	X
Energy	X	X	X
Calcium	X	X	X
Magnesium	X	X	X
Zinc	X	X	X
Copper	X	X	X
Selenium	X	?	
Iron		X	X
Vitamin A	X	X	X
Vitamin D	X	X	X
Vitamin E		X	X

may prioritize the immune system response over other maintenance requirements and become hypothermic. Metabolism may also be adversely impacted [4]. The cost of maintaining this state of immunological readiness is rarely considered. Investment in non-acute immune function is optional and sensitive to energetic resources and demands [5].

Furthermore, mounting an immune response against pathogens is an energetically demanding process. The immune system, in its responses to pathogens, must initiate leukocyte proliferation, antibody and cytokine production, and rapid increases in acute-phase proteins. These types of immune defenses are known to be energetically costly. Pyrogenic and non-febrile immune responses are associated with approximately 10% increases in metabolic rate [6, 7], and acute immune responses are associated with reductions in activity, body mass, and reproductive success in a wide range of animals [8].

How Do Macro Minerals Affect Immune System Function?

Minerals fulfill a wide variety of functions in the optimal functioning of the immune system. Both the innate defense system and the adaptive immune response are impacted by mineral levels in the body. Accordingly, the supply of minerals can influence susceptibility to infections, but it also has effects on the development of chronic diseases.

Calcium

Calcium (Ca^{2+}) acts as a necessary messenger in many cell types, including lymphocytes and phagocytic cells. Resting lymphocytes maintain a low concentration of Ca^{2+}. However, engagement of antigen receptors induces calcium influx from the extracellular space by several routes. Calcium signaling is also of paramount importance to immunity. Regulated increases in cytosolic and organellar Ca^{2+} concentrations in lymphocytes control complex and crucial effector functions such as metabolism, proliferation, differentiation, antibody and cytokine secretion, and cytotoxicity. Altered Ca^{2+} regulation in lymphocytes leads to various autoimmune, inflammatory, and immunodeficiency syndromes [9]. All phagocytic processes are regulated by a finely controlled rearrangement of the cell, where calcium (Ca^{2+}) signals play important roles. Ca^{2+} also affects the actions of many contractile proteins and serves as a cofactor in the activation of intracellular signaling proteins, known to play important roles during phagocytosis. In the mammalian immune system, Ca^{2+} is needed for the initial steps in phagocytosis and the subsequent phagosome maturation [10]. Calcium is also a second messenger that controls multiple processes in immune cells, including chemotaxis, adhesion, oxidative burst of phagocytic cells, and the secretion of pro- and anti-inflammatory cytokines [11].

Magnesium

Magnesium (Mg) has numerous roles in the regulation of immunological functions. This mineral influences the acute phase response and how macrophages respond to cytokines. Mg has a major influence on the development, differentiation, and proliferation of lymphocytes [12]. A Mg2+ transporter (TRPM7) has a special role in the development of T cells. In cells lacking this transporter, and thus an inadequate intracellular Mg supply, developmental inhibition and early cell death occurred [13]. Therefore, T-cell function is dependent on an adequate supply of Mg, both at the level of the individual cell and regarding the T-cell pool of an individual.

Mg deficiency stimulates an overfunction of the innate immune defense, with simultaneous deficiency of the adaptive immune defense. Mg deficiency has been demonstrated to increase aggregation of platelets, which impacts microvascular function. Experimental hypomagnesemia also disrupted Ca^{2+} homeostasis, which enhanced the pro-inflammatory effect of Mg deficiency [14]. There is evidence that the microbiota is also affected by systemic Mg deficiency. In this deficiency state, the concentration of bacteria in the intestine was reduced, while the barrier function of the intestinal wall was disturbed, which led to increased expression of tumor necrosis factor-α and interleukin (IL)-6 in the intestine and liver [15].

What Micro-minerals Are Necessary for Proper Immunity in Cattle?

Zinc

Zinc (Zn) is one of the trace minerals with a broader range of influences in the animal body. It participates in the structure and function of more than 2500 enzymes involved in metabolism, DNA replication, and the immune system [16]. Zinc is important in several aspects of the immune response, including participation in the proliferation and differentiation of lymphocytes, function and transit of neutrophils and macrophages, pro-inflammatory cytokines' production, regulation, and secretion (specifically IL-2), T-cell clonal expansion, and activation and antibody production by the B-cells [17].

Zn also acts as an antioxidant and influences the stability of biological membranes such as the T-cell receptor. A significant role is attributed to the trace element in the maintenance of immune homeostasis [18]. It affects the functional capacity of cells in the innate and adaptive immune system and has a regulatory effect on the production of cytokines, the activity of the complement system, and antibody production [19–21]. A deficiency of this element can contribute to a disturbance in immune function and thus have a significant impact on health. In vivo studies have also shown that Zn deficiency induces reduced adhesion and chemotaxis of monocytes and granulocytes, as well as impaired macrophage maturation and activity with reduced killing ability [22]. Zn also has a significant role in natural killer (NK) cells. Zn deficiency can induce a reduced NK cell count in the peripheral blood and lead to impaired functionality that include reduced chemotaxis, and lysis of virus-infected cells or tumor cells [12]. Zn has an important influence on the formation, maturation, and function of T cells [18]. It has been shown that Zn deficiency can result in a reduced ability in T-cell proliferation and cytokine production. Another significant role of Zn is that it is also important in T-cell differentiation processes [23]. Studies that induced Zn deficiency showed a reduction in the number of CD4+ T cells, with Th1 cells most impacted. Thus, Zn has a significant influence on viral infections, and it can positively influence, or even prevent, the course of disease.

In addition to its effect on selective immune functions, Zn status is associated with the overall regulation of the immune system. Studies show that, in addition to adapted immune system activation, increased oxidative stress and systemic inflammatory responses are induced by Zn deficiency [24–26]. Zn can influence both the production and the signaling of numerous inflammatory cytokines.

These studies highlight the importance of Zn for immune function, but there are also conflicting results showing that high doses of Zn cause immune dysfunction and associated health problems [12].

Copper

Copper (Cu) in the body is very sensitively balanced, as Cu in small amounts is necessary for many physiological processes, but too much Cu can be very harmful. Among the micronutrients in the serum, Cu is involved with systemic immune activity [27]. Copper is important in mitochondrial energy production and plays an essential role in neutralizing reactive oxygen species (ROS). The phagocyte killing activity and functions of neutrophils and monocytes, which are of high importance in the innate immune response of cattle, also depend on copper [28]. With regard to the adaptive arm of the immune system, defective antibody production and lowered cell-mediated immunity are associated with copper deficiency in mice [29].

Cu deficiency can lead to reduced humoral and cellular immune function. There is also neutropenia and lowered numbers of T cells. Mitogen-induced T-cell proliferation is impaired, as is the function of B cells and NK cells [30, 31]. Cu may also have anti-viral activities that can serve preventively and therapeutically [32]. Cu intake should be well balanced, as small amounts are sufficient for optimal immune function, while too much can have harmful effects at the same time [33].

Selenium

Selenium (Se) is an essential trace element that maintains homeostasis in humans and animals. Adequate selenium is essential for immune system function. Individual selenoproteins regulate inflammation and immunity. Se levels can also affect antiviral immunity, autoimmunity, sepsis, allergic asthma, and chronic inflammatory disorders [34].

Even marginal selenium deficiency can cause subclinical effects in cattle and strongly influence the immune system. The function of selenium in the immune system is based on its participation in the structure and function of several enzymes directly linked to the neutralization of ROS. Among them, glutathione peroxidase is a major antioxidant that reduces the excessive ROS and cell damage due to oxidative stress [35, 36]. Se deficiency in cattle may also increase the pathogenicity of some viruses [37] and decrease neutrophil migration into tissues that experience inflammation [38]. In contrast, providing Se supplementation enhances antibody production and T-cell number and functions [39].

Interestingly, selenium supplementation in subjects with low plasma Se improved T-cell-mediated immune responses to an oral vaccine and has been seen to result in more rapid clearance of the poliovirus and a reduced number of viral mutations [40].

Recent studies have shown that selenium deficiency can activate increased inflammatory cytokines. This inflammation was found to be mediated by heat shock proteins [41].

While Se is essential for maintaining the efficient function of the immune system, it is also possible for excessive amounts of Se to have adverse effects in cattle that already have adequate Se status.

Iron

Iron (Fe) is used in immune system development and function. Fe deficiency has been shown to decrease B-cell proliferation, T-lymphocyte function, and antibody responses [42, 43]. However, the indiscriminate use of Fe supplements in developing countries increased morbidity and mortality from health issues, including diarrhea. It is thought that these issues arise from an increase in Fe availability, which is used by the invading pathogens to proliferate and survive.

In summary, it appears that maintaining a healthy Fe status is beneficial to ensure optimal immunocompetence. However, it is also clear that the body's innate and immediate response to infection is to restrict extracellular Fe availability, which limits the impact of the host feeding and decreases propagation of the pathogen.

Are Vitamins Involved in Immune Responses in Cattle?

Vitamin A

Vitamin A is a fat-soluble vitamin that can impact immune function. β-Carotene is the major precursor of vitamin A that occurs naturally in feedstuffs. β-carotene may affect immune function since it can serve as an antioxidant. Vitamin A-deficient animals are more susceptible to bacterial, viral, and parasitic infections [44]. β-Carotene and vitamin A enhance lymphocyte proliferation and mitogen-induced blastogenesis [45]. Vitamin A also aids in antibody production (IgG, IgE, and IgA) [46, 47]. Vitamin A deficiency leads to decreased local immunity [47]. Vitamin A also has an influence on phagocytic cells, increasing phagocytic activity [48].

Vitamin D

In addition to the important role vitamin D has in calcium absorption, vitamin D directly impacts the immune system. Vitamin D signaling has important implications regarding immune function and infectious disease resistance in cattle [49–52]. Vitamin D is a regulator of innate and adaptive immunity in cattle [50, 52, 53] and responses of monocytes activated via Toll-like receptor 4 [52].

However, vitamin D inhibits interferon-γ and IL-17 responses of antigen-specific T cells in culture [50] and proliferation of CD4+ and γδTCR+ T cells in cattle [54]. It is not clear how vitamin D affects protection (particularly anti-viral) with these adaptive immune system impacts.

Vitamin E

Selenium and vitamin E are usually discussed together due to the interactions between the two micronutrients in body functions. Both vitamin E and selenium are involved in the cellular antioxidant defense system. Vitamin E functions as an antioxidant that scavenges free radicals. The role of vitamin E as an antioxidant is an important component of its involvement in immune responses [55]. Vitamin E increases blood neutrophil bactericidal activity [56], IL-1 production, and major histocompatibility class II antigen expression by blood monocytes [57]. Vitamin E also improves lymphocyte blastogenic responses to PHA in young calves [58, 59]. Humoral immune response has been enhanced by increasing dietary vitamin E, and antibody responses have been more consistent [60].

Are There Other Nutritional Factors to Consider That Impact the Immune System of Cattle?

The least understood but perhaps the most critical impact of nutrition on ruminant health and immunity is rumen/gastrointestinal (GI) health. A healthy rumen with normal balanced microbiota not only provides essential nutrients for growth and immunity but also preserves the health of its host by destroying harmful byproducts of fermentation [61]. Nutritional diseases such as acidosis (subclinical or acute) can lead to a variety of disease processes, including metabolic diseases, autoimmune diseases, tumors, and inflammatory diseases. During digestive upsets, intestinal bacteria and their metabolites can migrate out of the GI tract (GIT) to other organs such as the mammary gland, lung, liver, uterus, and brain, leading to related diseases [62]. A second mechanism for impacting the immune system, during digestive upset, is the creation and release of endotoxin (lipopolysaccharides) and other toxic bacterial metabolites into the circulation of the animal [62–64]. The bovine lung is one of the target organs for circulating endotoxin, and pulmonary responses to endotoxin, including pulmonary edema, are higher than in many other species [65]. The effect of endotoxin in cattle is described in adverse reactions to vaccination in Chap. 14.

What Is GI Microbiota?

It is hard to decide if the *intestinal microbiome* should be under innate immunity or nutrition (Chap. 6). This critical component of ruminant physiology is involved in providing key nutrients, utilized by the immune system, as well as protecting the digestive system from foreign invaders [66]. The complex microbial community that resides in the ruminant GIT (rumen and lower digestive tract) is a crucial contributor to the maintenance of intestinal homeostasis, mucosal and lymphoid structure development, and activation of the host immune cell repertoire [67]. The rumen is a fermentation chamber that contains microorganisms that utilize plant-origin cellulose as a nutrient. The rumen microbiome is comprised of a high-density population of bacteria, archaea, ciliate protozoa, fungi, bacteriophage, and viruses [68]. The ruminant microbiome (rumen and lower GIT) provides protein, energy, and essential amino acids and vitamins, both from the digestion of cellulose and from the utilization of the microorganisms themselves as nutrients [66, 68]. The GIT may also directly stimulate immune responses, particularly in the GI mucosal immune system [69–71].

Conclusion

Nutrition plays a vital role in proper immune system function. The amount of nutrients needed for immunoenhancement is higher than the required amounts suggested by National Research Council [72]. However, caution must be exercised so that supplementation does not lead to toxic levels of the nutrients, as many have toxic side effects in cattle at higher levels. Furthermore, the source, storage, and type of nutrient can affect the levels dramatically. Testing animals for proper levels of these nutrients in serum, whole blood, and liver biopsy can ensure that cattle are absorbing proper amounts of key nutrients from their feed.

Your Case

History

A 1000 dairy heifer calf rearing facility in Minnesota switched from raising Holstein calves to Jersey calves in the late spring. The facility raised calves from 1 day of age to 4 months of age, at which time they were sent back to the dairy of origin. Approximately 3 months after the switch in calf breeds, the facility began experiencing an increased level of neonatal scours and pneumonia with increasing death loss. As colder weather approached, morbidity approached 100% (for diarrhea and/or pneumonia), and death loss increased to approximately 30%.

Pertinent Background Information

Oral modified live rotavirus/coronavirus vaccine is administered to each calf 20 min prior to colostrum feeding. Calves are given three quarts of colostrum;

total proteins consistently are above 5.9 mg/mL. Calves are transported every other day to the calf ranch (approximately 90 miles).

Neonatal diarrhea is first seen between 7 and 21 days of age, and respiratory disease between 4 and 7 weeks of age. Most mortality occurs between 3 and 7 weeks of age. Calves are housed in a converted farrowing barn with individual calf hutches. Hutches are bedded with straw. Weaning is completed at 8 weeks of age. Deep pharyngeal swabs are positive for bovine coronavirus (3/10), *Pasteurella multocida* (8/10), and *Mannheimia haemolytica* (5/10). Samples from intestinal samples included rotavirus, coronavirus, *E. coli, Salmonella* sp., and cryptosporia.

Questions for You

1. Which result is misleading?
2. What is the primary problem?
3. What would you look for to confirm your diagnosis?

Additional Readings

1. Munteanu C, Schwartz B. The relationship between nutrition and the immune system. Front Nutr. 2022;9:1082500. https://doi.org/10.3389/fnut.2022.1082500. PMID: 36570149; PMCID: PMC9772031.
2. Marcos A, Nova E, Montero A. Changes in the immune system are conditioned by nutrition. Eur J Clin Nutr. 2003;57(Suppl 1):S66–9. https://doi.org/10.1038/sj.ejcn.1601819.
3. Godden SM, Fetrow JP, Feirtag JM, Green LR, Wells SJ. Economic analysis of feeding pasteurized nonsaleable milk versus conventional milk replacer to dairy calves. J Am Vet Med Assoc. 2005;226:1547–54.
4. Bird L. Getting enough energy for immunity. Nat Rev Immunol. 2019;19:269. https://doi.org/10.1038/s41577-019-0159-y.
5. Shattuck-Heidorn H, Reiches MW, Prentice AM, Moore SE, Ellison PT. Energetics and the immune system: Trade-offs associated with non-acute levels of CRP in adolescent Gambian girls. Evol Med Public Health. 2017:27–38. https://doi.org/10.1093/emph/eow034. Epub 2016 Dec 21. PMID: 28003312; PMCID: PMC5381351.
6. Dubois E. The basal metabolism in fever. JAMA. 1922;77:352–7.
7. Muehlenbein M, Hirschtick J, Bonner J, Swartz AM. Toward quantifying the usage costs of human immunity: altered metabolic rates and hormone levels during acute immune activation in men. Am J Hum Biol. 2010;4:546–56.
8. Lochmiller R, Deerenberg C. Tradeoffs in evolutionary immunology: just what is the cost of immunity? Oikos. 2000;88:87–98.
9. Trebak M, Kinet JP. Calcium signalling in T cells. Nat Rev Immunol. 2019;19:154–69. https://doi.org/10.1038/s41577-018-0110-7.
10. Melendez AJ. Calcium signaling during phagocytosis. In: Madame curie bioscience database [Internet]. Austin: Landes Bioscience; 2000–2013. Available from: https://www.ncbi.nlm.nih.gov/books/NBK5971/.
11. Nunes P, Demaurex N. The role of calcium signaling in phagocytosis. J Leukoc Biol. 2010;88(1):57–68. https://doi.org/10.1189/jlb.0110028. Epub 2010 Apr 16. PMID: 20400677.

12. Weyh C, Krüger K, Peeling P, Castell L. The role of minerals in the optimal functioning of the immune system. Nutrients. 2022;14(3):644. https://doi.org/10.3390/nu14030644. PMID: 35277003; PMCID: PMC8840645.
13. Schmitz C, Perraud AL, Johnson CO, Inabe K, Smith MK, Penner R, Kurosaki T, Fleig A, Scharenberg AM. Regulation of vertebrate cellular Mg2+ homeostasis by TRPM7. Cell. 2003;114:191–200. https://doi.org/10.1016/S0092-8674(03)00556-7.
14. Malpuech-Brugère C, Rock E, Astier C, Nowacki W, Mazur A. Rayssiguier Y exacerbated immune stress response during experimental magnesium deficiency results from abnormal cell calcium homeostasis. Life Sci. 1998;63:1815–22. https://doi.org/10.1016/S0024-3205(98)00455-X.
15. Pachikian BD, Neyrinck AM, Deldicque L, de Backer FC, Catry E, Dewulf EM, Sohet FM, Bindels LB, Everard A, Francaux M, Guiot Y, Cani PD, Delzenne NM. Changes in intestinal bifidobacteria levels are associated with the inflammatory response in magnesium-deficient mice. J Nutr. 2010;140:509–14. https://doi.org/10.3945/jn.109.117374.
16. Bittar JHJ, Palomares RA. A research-based summary on trace minerals for cattle VM245, one of a series of the Veterinary Medicine—Large Animal Clinical Sciences Department, UF/IFAS Extension. 2021. https://doi.org/10.32473/edis-VM245-2021.
17. Palomares RA, Hurley DJ, Bittar JHJ, Saliki JT, Woolums AR, Moliere F, Havenga LJ, Norton NA, Sigmund AJ, Barber CE, Berger ML, Clark MJ, Fratto MA. Effects of injectable trace minerals on humoral and cell-mediated immune responses to bovine viral diarrhea virus, bovine herpes virus 1 and bovine respiratory syncytial virus following Administration of a Modified-Live Virus Vaccine in dairy calves. Vet Immunol Immunopathol. 2016;178:88–98. https://doi.org/10.1016/j.vetimm.2016.07.003.
18. Prasad AS. Zinc in human health: effect of zinc on immune cells. Mol Med. 2008;14:353–7. https://doi.org/10.2119/2008-00033.Prasad.
19. Haase H, Rink L. Multiple impacts of zinc on immune function. Metallomics. 2014;6:1175–80. https://doi.org/10.1039/c3mt00353a.
20. Haase H, Rink L. Zinc signals and immune function. Biofactors. 2014;40:27–40. https://doi.org/10.1002/biof.1114.
21. Rink L, Haase H. Zinc homeostasis and immunity. Trends Immunol. 2007;28:1–4. https://doi.org/10.1016/j.it.2006.11.005.
22. Shankar AH, Prasad AS. Zinc and immune function: the biological basis of altered resistance to infection. Am J Clin Nutr. 1998;68:447S–63S. https://doi.org/10.1093/ajcn/68.2.447S.
23. Sheikh A, Shamsuzzaman S, Ahmad SM, Nasrin D, Nahar S, Alam MM, Al Tarique A, Begum YA, Qadri SS, Chowdhury MI, Saha A, Larson CP, Qadri F. Zinc influences innate immune responses in children with enterotoxigenic Escherichia coli-induced diarrhea. J Nutr. 2010;140:1049–56. https://doi.org/10.3945/jn.109.111492.
24. Gammoh NZ, Rink L. Zinc in infection and inflammation. Nutrients. 2017;9:624. https://doi.org/10.3390/nu9060624.
25. Wong CP, Dashner-Titus EJ, Alvarez SC, Chase TT, Hudson LG, Ho E. Zinc deficiency and arsenic exposure can act both independently or cooperatively to affect zinc status, oxidative stress, and inflammatory response. Biol Trace Elem Res. 2019;191:370–81. https://doi.org/10.1007/s12011-019-1631-z.
26. Wong CP, Rinaldi NA, Ho E. Zinc deficiency enhanced inflammatory response by increasing immune cell activation and inducing IL6 promoter demethylation. Mol Nutr Food Res. 2015;59:991–9. https://doi.org/10.1002/mnfr.201400761.
27. Malavolta M, Piacenza F, Basso A, Giacconi R, Costarelli L, Mocchegiani E. Serum copper to zinc ratio: relationship with aging and health status. Mech Ageing Dev. 2015;151:93–100. https://doi.org/10.1016/j.mad.2015.01.004.
28. Linder MC. Biochemistry of copper. In: Frieden E, editor. Biochemistry of the elements. New York: Plenum Press; 1991. https://doi.org/10.1007/978-1-4757-9432-8.
29. Sherman AR. Zinc, copper, and iron nutriture and immunity. In: History of nutritional immunology. 75th meeting of the Federation of American Societies for Experimental Biology, Atlanta, GA; 1992.

30. Kelley DS, Daudu PA, Taylor PC, Mackey BE, Turnlund JR. Effects of low-copper diets on human immune response. Am J Clin Nutr. 1995;62:412–6. https://doi.org/10.1093/ajcn/62.2.412.
31. Stabel JR, Spears JW. Effect of copper on immune function and disease resistance. Adv Exp Med Biol. 1989;258:243–52. https://doi.org/10.1007/978-1-4613-0537-8_22.
32. Raha S, Mallick R, Basak S, Duttaroy AK. Is copper beneficial for COVID-19 patients? Med Hypotheses. 2020;142:109814. https://doi.org/10.1016/j.mehy.2020.109814.
33. Besold AN, Culbertson EM, Culotta VC. The Yin and Yang of copper during infection. J Biol Inorg Chem. 2016;21:137–44. https://doi.org/10.1007/s00775-016-1335-1.
34. Huang Z, Rose AH, Hoffmann PR. The role of selenium in inflammation and immunity: from molecular mechanisms to therapeutic opportunities. Antioxid Redox Signal. 2012;16:705–43. https://doi.org/10.1089/ars.2011.4145.
35. Herdt TH, Hoff B. The use of blood analysis to evaluate trace mineral status in ruminant livestock. Vet Clin Food Anim. 2011;27:255–83. https://doi.org/10.1016/j.cvfa.2011.02.004.
36. Beck MA. Selenium and vitamin E status: impact on viral pathogenicity. J Nutr. 2007;37(5):1338–40. https://doi.org/10.1093/jn/137.5.1338.
37. Reeves MA, Hoffmann PR. The human selenoproteome: recent insights into functions and regulation. Cell Mol Life Sci. 2009;66:2457–78. https://doi.org/10.1007/s00018-009-0032-4.
38. Maddox JF, Aherne KM, Channa Reddy C, Sordillo LM. Increased neutrophil adherence and adhesion molecule mRNA expression in endothelial cells during selenium deficiency. J Leuk Biol. 1999;65:658–64. https://doi.org/10.1002/jlb.65.5.658.
39. Maggini S, Wintergerst ES, Beveridge S, Hornig DH. Elected vitamins and trace elements support immune function by strengthening epithelial barriers and cellular and humoral immune responses. Br J Nutr. 2007;98:S29–35. https://doi.org/10.1017/S0007114507832971.
40. Broome CS, McArdle F, Kyle JAM, Andrews F, Lowe NM, Hart CA, Arthur JR, Jackson MJ. An increase in selenium intake improves immune function and poliovirus handling in adults with marginal selenium status. Am J Clin Nutr. 2004;80:154–62. https://doi.org/10.1093/ajcn/80.1.154.
41. Zhang Y, Cui J, Lu Y, Huang C, Liu H, Xu S. Selenium deficiency induces inflammation via the iNOS/NF-κB pathway in the brain of pigs. Biol Trace Elem Res. 2020;196:103–9. https://doi.org/10.1007/s12011-019-01908-y.
42. Ward RJ, Crichton RR, Taylor DL, Della Corte L, Srai SK, Dexter DT. Iron and the immune system. J Neural Transm. 2011;118:315–28. https://doi.org/10.1007/s00702-010-0479-3.
43. Mullick S, Rusia U, Sikka M, Faridi MA. Impact of iron deficiency anaemia on T lymphocytes & their subsets in children. Indian J Med Res. 2006;124:647–54.
44. Scrimshaw NS, Taylor CE, Gordon JE. In interactions of nutrition and infection. World Health Org Monogr. 1968;57:87–94.
45. Chew BP. Immune function: relationship of nutrition and disease control. Vitamin a and beta-carotene on host defense. J Dairy Sci. 1987;70(12):2732–43. https://doi.org/10.3168/jds.s0022-0302(87)80346-6.
46. Jurin M, Tannock IF. Influence of vitamin a on immunological response. Immunology. 1972;23:283.
47. Sirisinha S, Darip MD, Moongkarndi P, Ongsakul M, Lamb AJ. Impaired local immune response in vitamin A-deficient rats. Clin Exp Immunol. 1980;40:127.
48. Moriguchi S, Werner L, Watson RR. High dietary vitamin A (retinyl palmitate) and cellular immune functions in mice. Immunology. 1985;56:169.
49. Lippolis JD, Reinhardt TA, Sacco RA, Nonnecke BJ, Nelson CD. Treatment of an intramammary bacterial infection with 25-hydroxyvitamin D3. PLoS One. 2011;6:e25479. https://doi.org/10.1371/journal.pone.0025479.
50. Nelson CD, Nonnecke BJ, Reinhardt TA, Waters WR, Beitz DC, Lippolis JD. Regulation of Mycobacterium-specific mononuclear cell responses by 25-hydroxyvitamin D3. PLoS One. 2011;6:6 10.1371/journal.pone.0021674.

51. Nelson CD, Reinhardt TA, Beitz DC, Lippolis JD. In vivo activation of the intracrine vitamin D pathway in innate immune cells and mammary tissue during a bacterial infection. PLoS One. 2010. 5 10.1371/journal.pone.0015469;5:e15469.
52. Nelson CD, Reinhardt TA, Thacker TC, Beitz DC, Lippolis JD. Modulation of the bovine innate immune response by production of 1alpha,25-dihydroxyvitamin D3 in bovine monocytes. J Dairy Sci. 2010;93:1041–9.
53. Nelson CD, Reinhardt TA, Lippolis JD, Sacco RE, Nonnecke BJ. Vitamin D signaling in the bovine immune system: a model for understanding human vitamin D requirements. Nutrients. 2012;4(3):181–96. https://doi.org/10.3390/nu4030181. Epub 2012 Mar 15. PMID: 22666545; PMCID: PMC3347026.
54. Waters WR, Nonnecke BJ, Foote MR, Maue AC, Rahner TE, Palmer MV, Whipple DL, Horst RL, Estes DM. Mycobacterium bovis bacille Calmette-Guerin vaccination of cattle: activation of bovine CD4+ and gamma delta TCR+ cells and modulation by 1,25-dihydroxyvitamin D3. Tuberculosis (Edinb). 2003;83:287–97. https://doi.org/10.1016/S1472-9792(03)00002-7.
55. Bendich A. Biological functions of dietary carotenoids. Ann N Y Acad Sci. 1993;691:61–7. https://doi.org/10.1111/j.1749-6632.1993.tb26157.x.
56. Hogan JS, Smith KL, Weiss WP, Todhunter DA, Schockey WL. Relationships among vitamin E, selenium, and bovine blood neutrophils. J Dairy Sci. 1990;73(9):2372–8. https://doi.org/10.3168/jds.S0022-0302(90)78920-5.
57. Politis I, Hidiroglou M, Batra TR, Gilmore JA, Gorewit RC, Scherf H. Effects of vitamin E on immune function of dairy cows. Am J Vet Res. 1995;56(2):179–84.
58. Reddy PG, Morrill JL, Minocha HC, Morrill MB, Dayton AD, Frey RA. Effect of supplemental vitamin E on the immune system of calves. J Dairy Sci. 1986;69:164.
59. Garber MJ, Roeder RA, Davidson PM, Pumfrey WM, Schelling GT. Dose response effects of vitamin E supplementation on growth performance and meat characteristics in beef and dairy steers. Can J Anim Sci. 1996;76:63–72.
60. Finch JM, Turner RJ. Effects of selenium and vitamin E on the immune responses of domestic animals. Res Vet Sci. 1996;60(2):97–106.
61. Du Y, Gao Y, Hu M, Hou J, Yang L, Wang X, Du W, Liu J, Xu Q. Colonization and development of the gut microbiome in calves. J Anim Sci Biotechnol. 2023;14(1):46. https://doi.org/10.1186/s40104-023-00856-x. PMID: 37031166; PMCID: PMC10082981.
62. Fu Y, He Y, Xiang K, Zhao C, He Z, Qiu M, Hu X, Zhang N. The role of rumen microbiota and its metabolites in subacute ruminal acidosis (SARA)-induced inflammatory diseases of ruminants. Microorganisms. 2022;10(8):1495. https://doi.org/10.3390/microorganisms10081495. PMID: 35893553; PMCID: PMC9332062.
63. Plaizier JC, Li S, Le Sciellour M, Schurmann BL, Górka P, Penner GB. Effects of duration of moderate increases in grain feeding on endotoxins in the digestive tract and acute phase proteins in peripheral blood of yearling calves. J Dairy Sci. 2014;97:7076–84. https://doi.org/10.3168/jds.2014-8162.
64. Monteiro HF, Faciola AP. Ruminal acidosis, bacterial changes, and lipopolysaccharides. J Anim Sci. 2020;98(8):skaa248. https://doi.org/10.1093/jas/skaa248. PMID: 32761212; PMCID: PMC7455920.
65. Templeton CB, Bottoms GD, Fessler JF, Turek JJ. Hemodynamics, plasma eicosanoid concentrations, and plasma biochemical changes in calves given multiple injections of Escherichia coli endotoxin. Am J Vet Res. 1988;49:90–5.
66. Malmuthuge N, Guan LL. Understanding host-microbial interactions in rumen: searching the best opportunity for microbiota manipulation. J Anim Sci Biotechnol. 2017;8:8.
67. Francino MP. Early development of the gut microbiota and immune health. Pathogens. 2014;3:769–90. https://doi.org/10.3390/pathogens3030769.
68. Mccann JC, Wickersham TA, Loor JJ. High-throughput methods redefine the rumen microbiome and its relationship with nutrition and metabolism. Bioinform Biol Insights. 2014;8:109–25.

69. Malmuthuge N, Liang G, Griebel PJ, Guan LL. Taxonomic and functional compositions of the small intestinal microbiome in neonatal calves provide a framework for understanding early life gut health. Appl Environ Microbiol. 2019;85:6e02534–18.
70. O'Hara E, Neves ALA, Song Y, Guan LL. The role of the gut microbiome in cattle production and health: driver or passenger? Annu Rev Anim Biosci. 2020;8:199–220. https://doi.org/10.1146/annurev-animal-021419.
71. Liang G, Malmuthuge N, Guan LL, Griebel P. Model systems to analyze the role of miRNAs and commensal microflora in bovine mucosal immune system development. Mol Immunol. 2015;66(1):57–67.
72. Nockels CN. Antioxidants improve cattle immunity following stress. Anim Feed Sci Technol. 1996;62(1):59–68. https://doi.org/10.1016/S0377-8401(96)01006-1. ISSN 0377-8401.

Bovine Parasites and Immunology

9

Abstract

For much of the world, control of internal and external parasites is as, or even more, important than controlling infectious diseases. Cattle parasites can severely affect production, overall health, and even cause direct death loss. They are also involved in transmitting other diseases, and some parasites have direct immunosuppressive activity. Immune responses against parasites are often complex, incomplete, and non-protective. However, immunologic research continues to be performed, as vaccination may provide a long-term solution to controlling many of these parasites.

Keywords

Internal parasites · External parasites · Lice · Ticks · Flies · Tapeworms · Coccidia · Cryptosporidium · Giardia · Trichostrongyles

Key Concepts

- Globally, internal and external parasites represent significant costs in cattle production.
- Parasitic infection can affect production and health. If severe enough, they may need to lead to death.
- Parasites in cattle are divided into internal and external parasites.
- While immune responses are stimulated during parasitic infections, effective vaccines have not been developed.

J. Ellis, V. Cortese, *Practical Bovine Immunology*,
https://doi.org/10.1007/978-3-032-15031-8_9

Why Are Parasites Important?

Internal and external parasites have a tremendous impact on cattle health and performance. Parasitic infections cause losses well exceeding US$21 billion per year [1]. This impact is seen in cattle-producing areas throughout the world; for example, ticks affect 80% of the world's cattle [1]. In its broadest definition, a parasite is any organism living in, on, or with another organism in order to obtain nutrients, grow, or multiply, often in a state that directly or indirectly harms the host. This broad definition would include bacteria and viruses. However, most consider parasites to be a pathogen that undergoes a life cycle that includes different forms. Viruses are different and require a cellular host to replicate their DNA or RNA genomes within cells. Depending on their structure, they can survive outside of a host for variable periods of time, but cannot replicate there. Bacteria are typically larger and single-celled, walled organisms, usually with a single circular DNA molecule, usually DNA encased by a cell membrane. Bacteria can also survive, and many can replicate outside cells in various environments. In contrast, the parasites we generally think of are mostly larger and more complex than bacteria. They live on or in a host organism and require a host for survival for at least part of their often-complex life cycle. Different stages of parasite life cycles can present varied immunologic targets, making protection difficult to obtain. Bovine parasites can have negative effects that include subclinical immune suppression, irritation, annoyance, appetite suppression, and decreased production, to severe clinical disease and death. This chapter will focus on the following parasites:

1. *Protozoa* are single-celled organisms that can spread through contaminated food, the environment, and some by insect vectors
2. *Metazoa* are multiple-celled organisms, usually with multiple-stage life cycles:
    A. Helminths are parasitic worms, the majority of which are gastrointestinal (GI) invaders.
    B. Ectoparasites are parasites that live on the outside of the body. These include ticks, flies, and lice.

What Are the Major Protozoal Infections of Cattle?

Protozoa are single-celled organisms, of which over 65,000 species have been described. The majority occur as either free-living forms or harmless commensals. Ruminants carry large numbers of protozoa in their stomachs and intestines, the vast majority of which are entirely harmless [1]. These protozoa play a vital role in controlling the bacterial population and biomass [2].

Some species of protozoa can cause significant disease in cattle, and many have potential for zoonotic transmission and cause disease in humans.

While some of these protozoa (Eimeria, Cryptospordia, and Giardia) are found in contaminated and/or aqueous environments and the soil, others are transmitted to cattle through an intermediate or primary host. The most common pathogenic protozoa of cattle are listed in Table 9.1.

What Type of Immune Response Do Cattle Have Against GI Protozoal Infections?

The immune response against the protozoal invaders will vary by the species, method of transmission, and sites of infection. The GI protozoal (Eimeria, Cryptospordia, and Giardia) exposures occur due to uptake of the protozoa from contaminated feed, water, and soil. While animals of all ages are susceptible to infection, younger animals are generally more susceptible to disease. Colostrum provides some passive immunity against GI protozoa during the first few weeks of life. Susceptibility can increase as maternal antibodies degrade. Severity of infection is usually related to the amount of environmental contamination and/or poor colostrum transfer. In older calves and adults, overcrowding, stress, or poor nutrition can increase the likelihood of an outbreak, particularly of coccidia.

GI protozoal infections stimulate both cellular and humoral immune responses. High IgM, IgG, and IgA antibody titers are seen following an infection [3]. However, antigen-specific humoral immune responses cannot eliminate primary infection [4–6] and are not protective against infections [5–7]. Since humoral immunity is not protective, newer studies have shown that T cells play the primary role in protective immunity against GI protozoa. T-cell mediated immune responses involve primarily CD4+ (primarily Th1), γδ T cells, and CD8+ lymphocytes [5–9]. T cell activation increases the levels of certain cytokines (such as interleukin (IL)2, IL4, and IFN-γ), activating the migration of immune cells to the site of infection [5, 6, 10–15]. Recently, IL17 has been shown to recruit immune cells to the site of infection in response to GI protozoal infections [5, 6, 11]. Even though infection with Eimeria and Cryptosporidia induces protective immunity that is long-lasting and specific to that particular parasite, no effective cattle vaccines have been developed [16]. Giardia vaccine development has also been unsuccessful [17].

What About Immune Responses to Vector/Intermediate Host Protozoal Infections?

The immune responses, against many of the systemic protozoal infections, are unclear and usually not protective. Many of the systemic protozoal infections can lead to persistent infection (Babesia and Neospora) [18, 19] or protected cysts (Besnoitia, Neospora, Sarcocystis, and Toxoplasma) [20–23]. This is further confounded by the fact that the life cycle and pathogenesis for some of these protozoa are not well understood [20]. If the infection in cattle involves several different stages of the protozoa, then the immune response may be different for each stage

Table 9.1 Most common protozoal infections in cattle. Not all are known to cause disease

Protozoa	Primary site of infection	Intermediate or primary host	Distribution
Babesia bigemina	Erythrocytes	Ticks	Americas, Europe, Africa, Australia, Middle East
Babesia bovis (*B. berbera*, *B. argentina*)	Erythrocytes	Ticks	Americas, Europe, Asia, Africa, Australia, Middle East, Russia
Babesia divergens	Erythrocytes	Ticks	Europe
Babesia major	Erythrocytes	Ticks	Europe, Russia, North Africa, Middle East
Babesia jakimovi	Erythrocytes	Ticks	Asia
Babesia ovata	Erythrocytes	Ticks	Japan
Besnoitia besnoiti	Skin, conjunctiva	Blood-feeding insects	Africa, Asia, Southern Europe
Cryptosporidium parvum	Small intestine	Contaminated environment	Worldwide
Cryptosporidium andersoni	Abomasum	Contaminated environment	Worldwide
Eimeria zuernii	Small and large intestine	Contaminated environment	Worldwide
Eimeria bovis	Small and large intestine	Contaminated environment	Worldwide
Eimeria auburnensis	Small intestine	Contaminated environment	Worldwide
Eimeria alabamensis	Small and large intestine	Contaminated environment	Worldwide
Eimeria bukidnonensis	?	Contaminated environment	Worldwide
Eimeria cylindrica	?	Contaminated environment	Worldwide
Eimeria canadensis	?	Contaminated environment	Worldwide
Eimeria ellipsoidalis	Small intestine	Contaminated environment	Worldwide
Eimeria pellita	?	Contaminated environment	Worldwide
Eimeria subspherica	?	Contaminated environment	Worldwide
Eimeria wyomingensis	?	Contaminated environment	Worldwide
Eimeria brasiliensis	?	Contaminated environment	Worldwide
Giardia intestinalis (*G. duodenalis* and *G. lambdia*)	Small intestine	Contaminated environment	Worldwide
Neospora caninum	Fetal infections	Dog	Worldwide
Sarcocystis bovicanis (cruzi)	Vascular endotheliun/ muscle	Dog	Worldwide

(continued)

Table 9.1 (continued)

Protozoa	Primary site of infection	Intermediate or primary host	Distribution
Sarcocystis bovifelis (hirsuta)	Vascular endotheliun/ muscle	Cat	Worldwide
Sarcocystis bovihominis (hominis)	Vascular endotheliun/ muscle	Human	Worldwide
Theileia annulata	Lymphocytes, erythrocytes	Tick	Mediterranean countries, Middle East, India, China
Theileia orientalis	Lymphocytes, erythrocytes	Tick	Southern Europe, Middle East, Australia, Asia
Theileia velifera	Lymphocytes, erythrocytes	Tick	Africa
Theileia taurotragi	Lymphocytes, erythrocytes	Tick	Africa
Theileia mutans	Lymphocytes, erythrocytes	Tick	Africa, Caribbean Islands
Toxoplasma gondii	Systemic	Cats	Worldwide
Trypanosoma brucei brucei	Systemic	Tsetse fly	Africa
Trypanosoma brucei evansi	Systemic	Blood-feeding insects	India
Trypanosoma congolense	Systemic	Tsetse fly	Africa
Trypanosoma vivax	Systemic	Tsetse fly	Africa
Trypanosoma theileri	Systemic	Blood-feeding insects	North America (worldwide?)

[24, 25]. Even though antigen-specific antibodies are present in the serum of immune animals, these antibodies are not protective for some of these protozoal infections (Theileria, Neospora, and Babesia) [19, 26–28]. However, antibodies may be important for protection against Toxoplasma [22, 29], Sarcocystis [30], and Trypanosomes [31–33]. For all of the non-GI protozoal infections, there is evidence that innate immunity (particularly phagocytic cells) and cell-mediated immunity and cytokine release are involved in the protection or survival of infected animals.

What Other Internal Parasites Are Important in Cattle?

All grazing animals become infected with non-protozoal GI parasites during their lifetime. The majority of parasites that infect the GI tract of ruminants are nematodes; occasionally, cestodes (tapeworms) may cause disease [34]. The severity of parasitic disease can range from subclinical to fatal disease, depending on the animals' immunity, the level of exposure, other stressors, nutritional status, and/or illness. For practical purposes, GI nematodes of ruminants can be divided into two major categories (Table 9.2):

Table 9.2 Nematodes and Cestodes of cattle

Name	Family	Primary location in cattle	Geographic Distribution
Paramphistomum cervi (cotylophoron, calicophoron, gigantocotyle)	Trematode (fluke)	Rumen	Worldwide
Haemonchus (contortus, placei, similus)	Trichostrongyle (strongyles)	Abomasum	Worldwide
Ostertagia ostertagi	Trichostrongyle	Abomasum	Worldwide
Trichostrongylus axei	Trichostrongyle	Abomasum	Worldwide
Mecistocirrus digitatus	Trichostrongyle	Abomasum	Sub-tropical and tropical areas
Cooperia (punctata, oncophora, pectinate, surnbata)	Trichostrongyle	Small intestine	Worldwide
Strongyloides papillosus	Strongylidae Nontrichostrongyle	Small intestine, lungs	Worldwide
Bunostomum phlebotomum	Nontrichostrongyle	Small intestine	Worldwide
Nematodirus (helvetianus, spathiger, filicollis, battus)	Trichostrongyle (strongyles)	Small intestine	Worldwide
Toxocara vitulorum	Nontrichostrongyle	Small intestine	Worldwide
Moniezia (benedeni, expansa)	Cestodes (tapeworms)	Small intestine	Worldwide
Taenia saginata (*Cysticercus bovis* larval form)	Cestodes (tapeworms)	Large intestine, muscle	Worldwide
Stilesia hepatica	Cestodes (tapeworms)	Liver (bile ducts)	Africa, Asia
Aonchotheca (Capillaria) bovis	Nontrichostrongyle	Small intestine	North America and Eurasia
Oesophagostomum (radiatum, venulosum, and columbianum)	Nontrichostrongyle	Large intestine	Worldwide
Chabertia ovina	Nontrichostrongyle	Large intestine	Worldwide
Trichuris ovis	Nontrichostrongyle	Large intestine	Worldwide
Fasciola hepatica	Trematode (fluke)	Liver	Worldwide
Fascioloides magna	Trematode (fluke)	Liver	North America and Europe
Dictyocaulus viviparus	Nontrichostrongyle	Lungs, GI tract	Worldwide

- Trichostrongyles parasites (order Strongylida, also known as strongyles) include numerous genera. While their adult location in the GI tract may vary, their life cycles are similar, with slight differences in the length of each stage or their preferred environmental temperature ranges. Life cycles of all the trichostrongyles are direct and rely on uptake by cattle on infected pastures to cause an infection [34]. For these reasons, their diagnosis, treatment, control, and prevention are very similar.
- Nontrichostrongyle parasites have unique life cycles. Flukes and tapeworms can be included in this category.

How Does Immunity to Trichostrongyles Occur After Grazing?

Since the life cycle is similar for the parasites in this category, the immune response, after infection, is the same across the different genera. After an exposure period of several months, ruminants slowly acquire protective immunity to GI nematodes but can still carry small amounts of the parasite and excrete eggs [35]. The main exception is Ostertagia, where immunity is not evident until the animals are more than 2 years old. While the entire immune response is not understood in trichistrongyles, the innate and adaptive immune responses are utilized to kill and/or remove the parasite and limit the severity of the disease. Once the larvae have invaded the GI mucosal tissues, damage to epithelial cells stimulates innate lymphoid cells and natural killer cells. Antigen-presenting cells such as dendritic cells and intestinal macrophages are stimulated to generate an immune response in co-regulation with complement fixation and mucus secretions to resist the primary infection [36]. Infections elicit very strong Th2-like responses predominated by high levels of IL4, IgG1, and IgE antibodies, and mast cells [35–37]. To control secondary infections, the specific adaptive immune mechanisms are triggered. Antigens are presented to the host in the draining lymph nodes after infection, and within the first 3–4 days of infection, these cells have left the nodes, entered the peripheral circulation, and have homed to tissues immediately surrounding the parasite, where the cells become established [35–38]. Th2 lymphocytes coordinate the humoral immune response, which secrete the main cytokine IL4, as well as other cytokines (IL3, IL5, IL9, IL10, and IL13) [35–37]. These cytokines stimulate eosinophils and mast cells. IgA and IgE are the most common antibodies at the mucosal sites of helminth infections. IgG is predominantly detected in the serum of infected animals [36]. For Ostertagia infections, the immune response elicited is not simply a stereotypic Th2 response. Different from other intestinal parasites, Ostertagia has evolved means to suppress or evade protective immune mechanisms. Despite all that is known about the immune response to Trichostrongyles, no vaccines have been developed yet against these intestinal parasites.

Is the Immune Response to Other Nematode Infections Similar to Immune Responses Against Trichostrongyle Infections?

While not as much detail is known about the immune responses against other GI nematode infections, several (Trichuris, Chabertia, Bunostomum, Oesophagostomum, Toxocara, and Anotheca) exhibit immune responses very similar to those seen against Trichostrongyles [36, 37, 39–41]. For lungworm infections (*Dictyocaulus viviparus*), antibodies confer little protection [42], and gamma delta T cells are more consistently stimulated during infection [43]. Like many nematodes, Dictyocaulus has the ability to down-regulate immune responses directed against the parasite [43–45]. Little research has been done on the immune response against *Strongyloides papillosus*, since there is a migratory phase to the lungs, and immune responses may be similar to lungworms [46].

Cestodes are invertebrate parasitic flatworms usually requiring one or two hosts for their transmission. They are generally considered nonpathogenic except in young calves or with overwhelming infection levels, where intestinal stasis, diarrhea, colic, and weight loss may be seen. During the initial stages of tapeworm infections, a Th1-type cellular immune response occurs. A Th2-type profile develops if the life cycle includes cyst formation (*Taenia saginata–Cysticercus bovis*) and growth [47, 48]. In tapeworm infection, the type of response associated with protection depends on the stage of the parasite and its location within the host. While a balance between Th1 and Th2 responses is optimal to control parasite load and minimize collateral damage, the Th2-type response is considered necessary for expulsion of adult tapeworms from the intestine [47].

Liver flukes (*Fasciola* spp.) are important parasites of ruminant livestock worldwide, causing considerable economic loss due to decreased weight gain, feed efficiency, milk production, and liver condemnations [49]. Even though there are detectable antibodies to fluke antigens following exposure [50], there is no evidence for a protective immune response to *Fasciola hepatica* and *Fascioloides magna*. Infected cattle decrease the habitat for feeding flukes, but this is not due to an immune response [51]. In untreated cattle, many liver flukes will die within 18 months of infection, though some can survive for more than 2 years [51].

What Are the Common External Parasites of Cattle?

The major external parasites that affect cattle include flies, grubs, lice, mosquitoes, ticks, and mites (Table 9.3). These external parasites feed on body tissues such as blood and skin, and in addition, they cause irritation and discomfort that result in reduced weight gain and decreased production. External parasites negatively impact cattle health not only by robbing cattle of required nutrients but also by increasing animal stress and because they are vectors for other diseases, such as anaplasmosis, theileriosis, and other tickborne diseases.

Can Cattle Have Immune Responses Against External Parasites?

The primary immune responses mounted against external parasites (particularly blood-feeding insects) are aimed at the salivary proteins. These proteins aid in digestion as well as acting as anti-coagulants for blood-feeding insects. However, in most external parasites, antibody responses to these proteins are not protective [51–57] but may decrease fly load or blood intake by feeding flies [58]. Increases in both IgG and IgE are seen after multiple bites. Eosinophilia develops, and eosinophil and mast cell infiltration surround the insect bites [59–61]. These may be involved in much of the local hypersensitivity seen after fly bites.

One notable difference is the immune responses to cattle grubs. While not actually blood-feeding flies, cattle grubs, or warbles are the larval stage of several flies.

Table 9.3 Common external parasites of cattle

Name	Family	Primary location/meal	Geographic distribution
External parasites—flies			
Horn flies	*Haematobia irritans*	Back and shoulders/blood meal	Worldwide
Face flies	*Musca auturnnalis*	Face/Mucous, saliva, wounds	North America
Stable flies	*Stomoxys calcitrans*	Legs/blood meals	Worldwide
Black flies (gnats)	*Simulium* sp.	Blood meals/no particular area	Worldwide
Deer flies	*Cbrysops* sp.	Blood meals/ no particular area	Worldwide
Tsetse flies	*Glossina* sp.	Blood meals/ no particular area	Africa
Screwworm flies	*Cochliomyia hominivorax*	Maggots attack wounds, moist tissue/no particular area	North and South America
Horse flies	*Tabanus* sp.	Blood meals/ no particular area	Worldwide
Northern cattle grub (bomb flies)	*Hypoderma bovis*	Tissue while migrating/eggs on legs, larva around the spinal cord	Worldwide
Common cattle grub (heel flies)	*Hypoderma lineatum*,	Tissue while migrating/eggs on legs larva around the esophagus	Worldwide
Warble fly	*Hypoderma sinense*	Tissue while migrating/Eggs on legs larva around the esophagus	China
Midges	*Culicoides* sp.	blood meals/no particular area	Worldwide
External parasites—other			
Mosquitos	*Culex* sp., *Aedes* sp., *Psoropbora* sp., *Anopheles* sp., and so on	Blood meals/no particular area	Worldwide
Mites	*Psoroptes* sp., *Sarcoptes* sp., *Cborioptes* sp., *Demodex* sp.	On or in skin/ hind legs, neck, head	Worldwide
Ticks	(*Dermacentor* sp., *Amblyomma* sp., *lxodes* sp., *Boopbilus* sp., and so on)	Blood meals/no particular area	Worldwide
Biting lice	*Bovicola bovis*	Hair, bits of skin, dried skin secretions, dried blood, or raw flesh around wounds/ head, ears, topline	Worldwide
Sucking lice	*Haematopinus eurysternus*, *H. quadripertusus*, *Linognathus vituli*, *Solenoptes capillatus*,	Blood meals/head, ears, topline	Worldwide

The larvae migrate from the animal's heel, where the eggs are deposited, to either the back or the esophagus of the animal. Following several infestations, most cattle become completely resistant to cattle grubs, and immune responses decrease the grub levels and survivability in the animal [62–64]. The immune response against grubs involves humoral, innate cellular, and cell-mediated responses with lymphocyte proliferation and several cytokines being released [62, 64–66].

Little is known about the immune responses formed by cattle in lice and mite infestations, although immune responses to these ecto-parasites appear to be similar [67–70]. The development of antibodies against lice and mites increased parasite numbers and topical lesions [68–70]. Infestations may also cause suppression of T-cell function [68]. Immune suppression of T cells is one of the predisposing factors for lice and mite outbreaks, so this suppression may also increase parasite numbers and local lesions.

Conclusion

Fundamental research continues to demonstrate the complexity of the immune response against bovine parasites. Researchers continue to search for methods of vaccination against parasites in cattle. While some vaccines have been evaluated, vaccines have been largely ineffective and still are not available. As a result, routine anti-parastic treatments and preventative measures are still considered to be the best option for controlling parasites and their associated diseases.

Your Case

History

The owner of an organic beef operation noticed that a group of 45 Angus and Angus cross replacement heifers were losing weight, and several had slightly loose manure. The heifers were 45 days postweaning and ranged in age from 6.5 to 8 months old. Cattle were weaned and placed in a small pasture after weaning and maintained there for 2 months for observation of pneumonia before being placed on a larger pasture.

Nutrition

Heifers were fed round bales of mixed alfalfa hay, a corn/soybean supplement that included trace minerals and vitamins (20% CP, fed three times per week), and trace mineral salt blocks in addition to the grass pasture. Heifers were not implanted, and monesin was not added to the ration. Water was from a well, and the trough was filled as it was emptied automatically.

Physical Examination

Cattle were underweight with rough hair coats. Several exhibited a "pot belly" appearance or bottle jaw. Several heifers were weak. While a few had "looser" manure, the majority had normal feces. Examination of weak calves had pale mucous membranes with slow capillary refill times. Temperatures were normal, and no other disease was detected.

Questions

1. What is your presumptive diagnosis?
2. What diagnostic tests do you perform?
3. What is your treatment plan?

Additional Readings

1. Taylor M. Protozoal disease in cattle and sheep. In Pract. 2000;22 https://doi.org/10.1136/inpract.22.10.604.
2. Sahinduran S. Protozoan diseases in farm ruminants. In: A bird's-eye view of veterinary medicine; 2012. Chapter 23. https://doi.org/10.5772/30251.
3. Matos L, del Carmen MM, Molina JM, Ferrer O, Rodríguez F, Pérez D, López AM, Martín S, Hermosilla C, Taubert A, Ruiz A. Humoral immune responses of experimentally Eimeria ninakholyakimovae-infected goat kids. Comp Immunol Microbiol Infect Dis. 2017;51:60–5. ISSN 0147-9571. https://doi.org/10.1016/j.cimid.2017.04.002.
4. Daugschies A, Najdrowski M. Eimeriosis in cattle: current understanding. J Vet Med B Infect Dis Vet Public Health. 2005;52:417–27. https://doi.org/10.1111/j.1439-0450.2005.00894.x. s
5. Taghi-Kilani R, Sekla L, Hayglass KT. The role of humoral immunity in Cryptosporidium spp. infection. Studies with B cell-depleted mice. J Immunol. 1990;145:1571–6.
6. Singer SM, Fink MY, Angelova VV. Recent insights into innate and adaptive immune responses to Giardia. Adv Parasitol. 2019;106:171–208. https://doi.org/10.1016/bs.apar.2019.07.004. Epub 2019 Aug 1. PMID: 31630758; PMCID: PMC7086480.
7. Yun CH, Lillehoj HS, Lillehoj EP. Intestinal immune responses to coccidiosis. Dev Comp Immunol. 2000;24(2–3):303–24. https://doi.org/10.1016/s0145-305x(99)00080-4.
8. Matos L, Muñoz MC, Molina JM, Rodríguez F, Pérez D, López AM, Hermosilla C, Taubert A, Ruiz A. Age-related immune response to experimental infection with Eimeria Ninakohlyakimovae in Goat Kids. Res Vet Sci. 2018;118:155–63. https://doi.org/10.1016/j.rvsc.2018.02.004. [PubMed] [CrossRef] [Google Scholar].
9. Abrahamsen MS, Lancto CA, Walcheck B, Layton W, Jutila MA. Localization of alpha/beta and gamma/delta T lymphocytes in Cryptosporidium parvum-infected tissues in naive and immune calves. Infect Immun. 1997;65:2428–33.
10. Sühwold A, Hermosilla C, Seeger T, Zahner H, Taubert A. T cell reactions of Eimeria bovis primary and challenge-infected calves. Parasitol Res. 2010;106:595–605. https://doi.org/10.1007/s00436-009-1705-5. [PubMed] [CrossRef] [Google Scholar].
11. Grit GH, Van Coppernolle S, Devriendt B, Geurden T, Dreesen L, Hope J, Vercruysse J, Cox E, Geldhof P, Claerebout E. Evaluation of cellular and humoral systemic immune response against Giardia duodenalis infection in cattle. Vet Parasitol. 2014;202(3–4):145–55. https://doi.org/10.1016/j.vetpar.2014.03.012. Epub 2014 Mar 20.
12. Lillehoj HS. Immune response during Coccidiosis in SC and FP chickens. I. In vitro assessment of T cell proliferation response to stage-specific parasite antigens. Vet Immunol Immunopathol. 1986;13:321–30. https://doi.org/10.1016/0165-2427(86)90025-5. [PubMed] [CrossRef] [Google Scholar].
13. Taubert A, Hermosilla C, Sühwold A, Zahner H. Antigen-induced cytokine production in lymphocytes of Eimeria bovis primary and challenge infected calves. Vet Immunol Immunopathol. 2008;126:309–20. https://doi.org/10.1016/j.vetimm.2008.09.003. [PubMed] [CrossRef] [Google Scholar].
14. de Graaf DC, Walravens K, Godfroid J, Peeters JE. A Cryptosporidium parvum oocyst low molecular mass fraction evokes a CD4+ T-cell-dependent IFN-gamma response in bovine peripheral blood mononuclear cell cultures. Int J Parasitol. 1998;28:1875–80.
15. Takeda K, Omata Y, Koyama T, Ohtani M, Kobayashi Y, Furuoka H, Matsui T, Maeda R, Saito A. Increase of Th1 type cytokine mRNA expression in peripheral blood lymphocytes of calves experimentally infected with Cryptosporidium parvum. Vet Parasitol. 2003;113:327–31.
16. Thomson S, Hamilton CA, Hope JC, Katzer F, Mabbott NA, Morrison LJ, Innes EA. Bovine cryptosporidiosis: impact, host-parasite interaction and control strategies. Vet Res. 2017;48(42) https://doi.org/10.1186/s13567-017-0447-0.
17. Uehlinger FD, O'Handley RM, Greenwood SJ, Guselle NJ, Gabor LJ, Van Velsen CM, Steuart RF, Barkema HW. Efficacy of vaccination in preventing giardiasis in calves. Vet Parasitol.

2007;146(1–2):182–8. https://doi.org/10.1016/j.vetpar.2007.01.013. Epub 2007 Mar 12. PMID: 17350765; PMCID: PMC7126623.

18. Brown WC, Norimine J, Knowles DP, Goff WL. Immune control of Babesia bovis infection. Vet Parasitol. 2006;138(1–2):75–87. https://doi.org/10.1016/j.vetpar.2006.01.041. Epub 2006 Feb 28.
19. Almería S, Serrano-Pérez B, López-Gatius F. Immune response in bovine neosporosis: protection or contribution to the pathogenesis of abortion. Microb Pathog. 2017;109:177–82. https://doi.org/10.1016/j.micpath.2017.05.042. Epub 2017 May 31.
20. Gollnick NS, Scharr JC, Schares G, Langenmayer MC. Natural Besnoitia besnoiti infections in cattle: chronology of disease progression. BMC Vet Res. 2015;11:35. https://doi.org/10.1186/s12917-015-0344-6. PMID: 25886463; PMCID: PMC4357170.
21. Gasbarre LC, Suter P, Fayer R. Humoral and cellular immune responses in cattle and sheep inoculated with Sarcocystis. Am J Vet Res. 1984;45(8):1592–6.
22. Dupont CD, Christian DA, Hunter CA. Immune response and immunopathology during toxoplasmosis. Semin Immunopathol. 2012;34(6):793–813. https://doi.org/10.1007/s00281-012-0339-3. Epub 2012 Sep 7. PMID: 22955326; PMCID: PMC3498595.
23. Haddad JP, Dohoo IR, VanLeewen JA. A review of Neospora caninum in dairy and beef cattle--a Canadian perspective. Can Vet J. 2005;46(3):230–43. PMID: 15884645; PMCID: PMC1082867.
24. Dobbelaere DA, Spooner PR, Barry WC, Irvin AD. Monoclonal antibody neutralizes the sporozoite stage of different Theileria parva stocks. Parasite Immunol. 1984;6(4):361–70. https://doi.org/10.1111/j.1365-3024.1984.tb00808.x.
25. Goddeeris BM, Morrison I, Taracha EL, McKeever DL. East coast fever (Theileria parva); cell-mediated immunity and protection. In: Goddeeris BML, Morrison WI, editors. Cell mediated immunity in ruminants. CRC press; 1994. p. 143–56.
26. Muhammed SI, Lauerman LH Jr, Johnson LW. Effect of humoral antibodies on the course of Theileria parva infection (East Coast fever) of cattle. Am J Vet Res. 1975;36(4 Pt.1):399–402.
27. Innes EA, Andrianarivo AG, Björkman C, Williams DJ, Conrad PA. Immune responses to Neospora caninum and prospects for vaccination. Trends Parasitol. 2002;18(11):497–504. https://doi.org/10.1016/s1471-4922(02)02372-3.
28. Brown WC, Norimine J, Knowles DP, Goff WL. Immune control of Babesia bovis infection. Vet Parasitol. 2006;138(1–2):75–87. https://doi.org/10.1016/j.vetpar.2006.01.041. ISSN 0304-4017. [PubMed] [CrossRef] [Google Scholar] [Ref list].
29. Johnson LL, Sayles PC. Deficient humoral responses underlie susceptibility to Toxoplasma gondii in CD4-deficient mice. Infect Immun. 2002;70(1):185–91. [PMC free article] [PubMed] [Google Scholar].
30. Ellison S, Witonsky S. Evidence that antibodies against recombinant SnSAG1 of Sarcocystis neurona merozoites are involved in infection and immunity in equine protozoal myeloencephalitis. Can J Vet Res. 2009;73(3):176–83. PMID: 19794889; PMCID: PMC2705071.
31. Taylor KA. Immune responses of cattle to African trypanosomes: protective or pathogenic? Int J Parasitol. 1998;28(2):219–40. https://doi.org/10.1016/s0020-7519(97)00154-9.
32. Morrison WI, Black SJ, Paris J, Hinson CA, Wells PW. Protective immunity and specificity of antibody responses elicited in cattle by irradiated Trypanosoma brucei. Par Immunol. 1982;4(6):395–407.
33. Akol GW, Murray M. Induction of protective immunity in cattle by tsetse-transmitted cloned isolates of Trypanosoma congolense. Ann Trop Med Parasitol. 1985;79(6):617–27. https://doi.org/10.1080/00034983.1985.11811969. PMID: 3834843.
34. Strydom T, Lavan RP, Torres S, Heaney K. The economic impact of parasitism from nematodes, trematodes and ticks on beef cattle production. Animals. 2023;13:1599. https://doi.org/10.3390/ani13101599.
35. Gasbarre LC, Leighton EA, Sonstegard T. Role of the bovine immune system and genome in resistance to gastrointestinal nematodes. Vet Parasitol. 2001;98(1–3):51–64. https://doi.org/10.1016/s0304-4017(01)00423-x.

36. McRae KM, Stear MJ, Good B, Keane OM. The host immune response to gastrointestinal nematode infection in sheep. Parasite Immunol. 2015;37:605–13. https://doi.org/10.1111/pim.12290. [PMC free article] [PubMed] [CrossRef] [Google Scholar] [Ref list].
37. Hendawy SHM. Immunity to gastrointestinal nematodes in ruminants: effector cell mechanisms and cytokines. J Parasit Dis. 2018;42(4):471–82. https://doi.org/10.1007/s12639-018-1023-x. Epub 2018 Aug 9. PMID: 30538343; PMCID: PMC6261135.
38. Bhat AH, Tak H, Malik IM, Ganai BA, Zehbi N. Trichostrongylosis: a zoonotic disease of small ruminants. J Helminthol. 2023;97:e26. https://doi.org/10.1017/S0022149X2300007X.
39. Darlan DM, Rozi MF, Yulfi H. Overview of immunological responses and immunomodulation properties of Trichuris sp.: prospects for better understanding Human Trichuriasis. Life (Basel). 2021;11(3):188. https://doi.org/10.3390/life11030188. PMID: 33673676; PMCID: PMC7997218.
40. Herd RP. Studies on the immune response of sheep to Chabertia ovina (Fabricius, 1788). Internat J Parasitol. 1971;1(3–4):265–74. ISSN 0020-7519. https://doi.org/10.1016/0020-7519(71)90029-4.
41. de Souza EM, Starke-Buzetti WA, Ferreira FP, Neves MF, Machado RZ. Humoral immune response of water buffalo monitored with three different antigens of Toxocara vitulorum. Vet Parasitol. 2004;122(1):67–78. https://doi.org/10.1016/j.vetpar.2004.03.013.
42. Kooyman FN, Yatsuda AP, Ploeger HW, Eysker M. Serum immunoglobulin E response in calves infected with the lungworm Dictyocaulus viviparus and its correlation with protection. Parasite Immunol. 2002;24(1):47–56. https://doi.org/10.1046/j.0141-9838.2001.00436.x.
43. Hagberg M. Immune cell responses to the Cattle Lungworm, Dictyocaulus viviparus. 2008. 37 Acta Universitatis agriculturae Sueciae, PhD dissertation ISSN 1652-6880, ISBN 978-91-85913-70-1.
44. Maizels RM, Balic A, Gomez-Escobar N, Nair M, Taylor MD, Allen JE. Helminth parasites--masters of regulation. Immunol Rev. 2004;201:89–116. https://doi.org/10.1111/j.0105-2896.2004.00191.x. [PubMed] [CrossRef] [Google Scholar].
45. Maizels RM, Yazdanbakhsh M. Immune regulation by helminth parasites: cellular and molecular mechanisms. Nat Rev Immunol. 2003;3:733–44. https://doi.org/10.1038/nri1183. [PubMed] [CrossRef] [Google Scholar].
46. Hamsborg SM, Ketzis J, Horii Y, Matthews JB. Strongyloides spp. infections of veterinary importance. Parasitol. 2017;144(3):274–84. https://doi.org/10.1017/S0031182016001116.
47. Ríos-Valencia DG, Ambrosio J, Tirado-Mendoza R, Carrero JC, Laclette JP. What about the cytoskeletal and related proteins of tapeworms in the host's immune response? an integrative overview. Pathogens. 2023;12(6):840. https://doi.org/10.3390/pathogens12060840. PMID: 37375530; PMCID: PMC10302083.
48. Terrazas L. The complex role of pro- and anti-inflammatory cytokines in cysticercosis: immunological lessons from experimental and natural hosts. Curr Top Med Chem. 2008;8:383–92. https://doi.org/10.2174/156802608783790848. [PubMed] [CrossRef] [Google Scholar].
49. Hayward AD, Skuce PJ, McNeilly TN. The influence of liver fluke infection on production in sheep and cattle: a meta-analysis. Internat J Parasitol. 2021;51(11):913–24. ISSN 0020-7519. https://doi.org/10.1016/j.ijpara.2021.02.006.
50. Charlier J, Duchateau L, Claerebout E, Williams D, Vercruysse J. Associations between anti-Fasciola hepatica antibody levels in bulk-tank milk samples and production parameters in dairy herds. Prev Vet Med. 2007;78(1):57–66. ISSN 0167-5877. https://doi.org/10.1016/j.prevetmed.2006.09.010.
51. Forbes A. Liver fluke infections in cattle and sheep. Livestock. 2017;22(5). Published Online: 13 Sep 2017. https://doi.org/10.12968/live.2017.22.5.250.
52. Kerlin RL, Allingham PG. Acquired immune response of cattle exposed to buffalo fly (Haematobia irritans exigua). Vet Parasitol. 1992;43(1–2):115–29. https://doi.org/10.1016/0304-4017(92)90054-d.
53. Somda MB, Bengaly Z, Dama E, Poinsignon A, Dayo G-K, Sidibe I, Remoue F, Sanon A, Bucheton B. First insights into the cattle serological response to tsetse salivary antigens: a

promising direct biomarker of exposure to tsetse bites. Vet Parasitol. 2013;197:332–40. https://doi.org/10.1016/j.vetpar.2013.05.018. PubMed Abstract | CrossRef Full Text | Google Scholar.
54. Swist S, Wilkerson M, Wyatt C, Broce A, Kanost M. Modulation of bovine lymphocyte response by salivary gland extracts of the stable fly, Stomoxys calcitrans (Diptera: Muscidae). J Med Entomol. 2002;39:900–7. https://doi.org/10.1603/0022-2585-39.6.900. PubMed Abstract | CrossRef Full Text | Google Scholar.
55. Vogt MB, Lahon A, Arya RP, Kneubehl AR, Spencer Clinton JL, Paust S, Rico-Hesse R. Mosquito saliva alone has profound effects on the human immune system. PLoS Negl Trop Dis. 2018;12(5):e0006439. https://doi.org/10.1371/journal.pntd.0006439. PMID: 29771921; PMCID: PMC5957326.
56. Ndawula C Jr. From bench to field: a guide to formulating and evaluating anti-tick vaccines delving beyond efficacy to effectiveness. Vaccines (Basel). 2021;9(10):1185. https://doi.org/10.3390/vaccines9101185. PMID: 34696291; PMCID: PMC8539545.
57. Breijo M, Pastro L, Rocha S, Ures X, Alonzo P, Santos M, Bolatto C, Fernández C, Meikle A. A natural cattle immune response against Horn Fly (Diptera: Muscidae) salivary antigens may regulate parasite blood intake. J Econ Entomol. 2016;109(4):1951–6. https://doi.org/10.1093/jee/tow133. Epub 2016 Jun 21. PMID: 27329632.
58. Abbas MN, Jmel MA, Mekki I, Dijkgraaf I, Kotsyfakis M. Recent advances in tick antigen discovery and anti-tick vaccine development. Int J Mol Sci. 2023;24(5):4969. https://doi.org/10.3390/ijms24054969.
59. Fortes d AF, Maha A, Clarissa T, Kelly H, Wilkerson Matthew D, Roseanne R, Ines L-N, Ellis Michael W, Claudio M, Saule N, Regis G, David TW, Turiansky George W, Marzena P, Fabiano O, Valenzuela Jesus G, Shaden K, Naomi A. Immune response profiles from humans experimentally exposed to Phlebotomus duboscqi bites. Front Immunol. 2024; https://doi.org/10.3389/fimmu.2024.1335307.
60. Peng Z, Beckett AN, Engler RJ, Hoffman DR, Ott NL, Simons FE. Immune responses to mosquito saliva in 14 individuals with acute systemic allergic reactions to mosquito bites. J Allergy Clin Immunol. 2004;114(5):1189–94. https://doi.org/10.1016/j.jaci.2004.08.014. Erratum in: J Allergy Clin Immunol. 2005 Feb;115(2):376.
61. Robbertse L, Richards SA, Maritz-Olivier C. Bovine immune factors underlying tick resistance: integration and future directions. Front Cell Infect Microbiol. 2017;7:522. https://doi.org/10.3389/fcimb.2017.00522. PMID: 29312898; PMCID: PMC5742187.
62. Colwell DD. Stage specific mortality and humoral immune responses during pulse and trickle infestations of the common cattle grub, Hypoderma lineatum (Diptera: Oestridae). Vet Parasitol. 2001;99(3):231–9. https://doi.org/10.1016/s0304-4017(01)00459-9.
63. Baron RW, Colwell DD. Enhanced resistance to cattle grub infestation (Hypoderma lineatum de Vill.) in calves immunized with purified hypodermin A, B and C plus monophosphoryl lipid A (MPL). Vet Parasitol. 1991;38(2–3):185–97. https://doi.org/10.1016/0304-4017(91)90128-i.
64. Colwell DD. Hidden antigens from third instar Hypoderma lineatum: impact of immunization on larval survival in artificial infestations. Vet Parasitol. 2011;175(3–4):313–9. https://doi.org/10.1016/j.vetpar.2010.10.013. Epub 2010 Oct 15.
65. Gingrich RE. Acquired resistance to Hypoderma lineatum: comparative immune response of resistant and susceptible cattle. Vet Parasitol. 1982;9(3-4):253–60. ISSN 0304–4017. https://doi.org/10.1016/0304-4017(82)90069-3.
66. Baron RW, Weintraub J. Lymphocyte responsiveness in cattle previously infested and uninfested with Hypoderma lineatum (de Vill.) and H. bovis (L.) (Diptera: Oestridae). Vet Parasitol. 1987;24(3–4):285–96. ISSN 0304-4017. https://doi.org/10.1016/0304-4017(87)90050-1.
67. Chen Z, Claerebout E, Chier K, Pardon B, Casaert S, De Wilde N, Duchateau L, Geldhof P, van Mol W. Dermal immune responses against Psoroptes ovis in two cattle breeds and effects of anti-inflammatory dexamethasone treatment on the development of psoroptic mange. Vet Res. 2021;52(1) https://doi.org/10.1186/s13567-020-00874-x.

68. Pruett JH, Guillot FS, Fisher WF. Humoral and cellular immunoresponsiveness of stanchioned cattle infested with Psoroptes ovis. Vet Parasitol. 1986;22(1–2):121–33. ISSN 0304-4017. https://doi.org/10.1016/0304-4017(86)90014-2.
69. Colwell DD, Himsl-Rayner C. Linognathus vituli (Anoplura: Linognathidae): population growth, dispersal and development of humoral immune responses in naïve calves following induced infestations. Vet Parasitol. 2002;108(3):237–46. ISSN 0304-4017.
70. Milnes AS, Bailey M, Knowles TG, Coles GC, Green LE, Day MJ. An immunohistochemical assessment of the cutaneous immune response to Louse infestation in cattle. J Comp Pathol. 2007;136(4):240–9. ISSN 0021-9975. https://doi.org/10.1016/j.jcpa.2007.02.007.

Reproductive Immunology

10

Abstract

The mucosal immune system of the reproductive tract is unique since it must not only be able to recognize and tolerate sperm during impregnation and the developing fetus, both of which have foreign protein markers. It must also be able to respond to a myriad of bacterial exposures and viral diseases. Studies are now showing the impact of the immune system on all components of the reproductive cycle, from follicular development to maintaining pregnancy. While many of these studies have been done in species other than cattle, they provide valuable insight into the influence the immune system has on reproduction in mammals.

Keywords

Reproduction · Sperm · Oocytes · Fetus · Infertility · Regulatory T cells (Treg) · Corpus luteum · Pregnancy · Placenta · Interferon tau

Key Concepts

- The reproductive immune system is unique in that it must respond to pathogens but tolerate sperm and the developing fetus.
- The immune system, in concert with reproductive hormones, maintains normal follicular and luteal development.
- Local immune responses are directly involved in the routine estrus cycle in cows.

Why Is Reproductive Immunology Important?

Despite improvements gained by genomic selection, infertility and embryonic wastage cause major economic loss in cattle production [1]. Once pregnancy is achieved, most pregnancy losses occur during early pregnancy. *Infertility and embryonic*

J. Ellis, V. Cortese, *Practical Bovine Immunology*,
https://doi.org/10.1007/978-3-032-15031-8_10

losses lead to decreased milk yields, slower genetic improvement, and increased expenses [1, 2]. This is further exacerbated by diseases of the reproductive system, such as metritis, endometritis, pyometra, and retained fetal membranes, which can also lead to infertility and increased culling rates [3–5]. *Tolerance of fetal tissue* by the maternal immune system (fetal tolerance) was initially compared to transplantation tolerance due to the paternal half of its genetic makeup and the intimate relationship between maternal and fetal tissues. However, fetal tolerance is different in that tissue grafting is not a normal immunologic phenomenon, whereas fetal and semen tolerance are required in cattle and other viviparous mammals. Rather than just tolerance, it appears that there is cooperation between the fetus and the maternal immune system to promote implantation, placentation, and fetal growth [6–8]. Abnormal immune function has been identified as one of the primary causes of infertility [8, 9]. Since reproduction is such an important part of cattle production, understanding the relationship between the immune system and proper reproductive function is critical.

Does the Immune System Affect Ovarian Function?

While the major influence on bovine ovarian function is hormonal via the hypothalamus–pituitary–ovary axis [9, 10], there is increasing evidence for immunologic involvement in the estrous cycle and initiation of pregnancy [8, 11–15]. Immune cell-derived cytokines can also impact the production of these hormones [12]. Furthermore, immune cell populations and cytokine release play an important role in ovarian function, as they regulate ovarian development, follicular maturation, ovulation, and the formation of the corpus luteum [8, 11–15].

Ovarian germline stem cells (OSCs) are epithelial cells found on the ovarian surface. OSCs can differentiate into oocytes and granulosa cells and originate from stem cells of the ovarian cortex [16]. Factors within the OSC niche control ovarian functions. Immune cells and their cytokines are part of these factors [17]. The OSC niche is established during early stages of fetal development and consists of ovarian monocyte-derived cells (MDCs), T cells, and vascular endothelial cells. In adults, the OSC niche contains MDCs (CD14+ MDC), activated MDCs, and T cells. The immune system plays an important role in the development of OCSs and primordial follicles in both the fetus and the adult [12, 16, 17].

How Does the Immune System Impact the Estrous Cycle of Cattle?

In addition to the impact of the immune system on *developing follicles* as described above, the immune system is involved in the various stages of the *estrous cycle* of cattle (Fig. 10.1). Ovulation is an inflammatory event as leukocytes (primarily neutrophils, macrophages, and lymphocytes) move into the ovulatory follicle and changes are seen in cytokine expression in both the theca and granulosa layers [8,

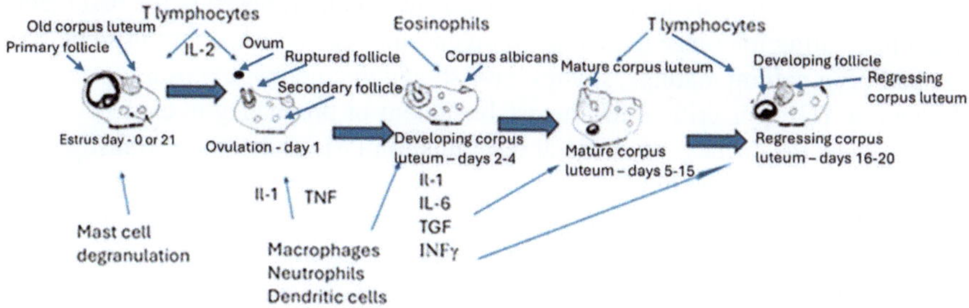

Fig. 10.1 Immune system interactions with the bovine ovary during the estrous cycle

11–15]. As follicles mature, increasing pressure causes the follicle to rupture, releasing the secondary oocyte. Cytokines (tumor necrosis factor (TNF)-α and IL-1) play an important role in both early and late stages of follicular development [13]. TNF-α promotes the secretion of Follicle Stimulating Hormone. These cytokines (particularly interleukin (IL)-1) can also inhibit prostaglandin F2α release, aiding in *ovulation* [18, 19]. The pre- and peri-ovulatory follicles also contain T-cells, neutrophils, macrophages, and dendritic cells. Dendritic cells are the most abundant cells in the ovulatory follicular and luteal tissue [8, 11]. In cattle, the Luteinizing Hormone in the ovulatory follicle stimulates a sterile inflammatory response, which resolves as the corpus luteum develops [11–21].

Leukocytes, with other ovarian cells, are involved in follicle repair and corpus luteum development by producing matrix metalloproteinases [22]. Cytokines, released by macrophages, specifically TNF and interferon gamma (and probably others), are active in the development and degeneration of the corpus luteum. There is an influx of T-lymphocytes just prior to the onset of luteolysis: 25% T helper cells (CD4+), 45% cytotoxic T-cells (CD8+), and 30% were gamma delta (γδ+) T-cells [23–25].

Cellular and cytokine interactions during the estrous cycle include cytokines released by lymphocytes, macrophages, dendritic cells, eosinophils, and mast cells, as well as direct cellular interactions.

Is the Immune System Involved in Fertilization and Impregnation of Cows?

Even though bovine semen enters the cervical canal quickly after breeding, the vaginal stimulation and seminal fluid (via transforming growth factor-beta (TGF-β), interferon gamma, and IL-8) attract neutrophils to the cervical and uterine tissues and stimulate the release of cytokines such as granulocyte-macrophage colony-stimulating factor [26–32]. These neutrophils specifically target non-motile or damaged spermatozoa [33–35]. Granulocytes may also be involved in clearing bacteria transmitted during the breeding process. The same responses may be seen with intrauterine horn insemination [36]. While this has been proposed as the first mechanism in creating tolerance to paternal antigens and may be important in some species and/or in natural matings, studies have shown that neither exposure to seminal plasma nor TGF-β is critical for the establishment of pregnancy in cattle [37, 38]. This explains the success of artificial insemination (AI) and embryo transfer (ET) programs where seminal fluid exposure does not occur.

The first exposure to paternal antigens in AI and ET programs occurs during embryo implantation [39]. The acceptance of paternal antigens cannot be explained by maternal immunosuppression or shifting of the immune response since cytokines are released during implantation [40–42]. While mechanisms may exist that prevent a maternal immune response against paternal antigens, the trophoblast and the maternal immune system establish a cooperative state [40, 43–47]. In ruminants, a unique type 1 interferon, interferon tau (IFN-τ), is secreted by trophoblasts and endometrial cells and is a signal for the maternal recognition of the pregnancy, thus maintaining corpus luteum progesterone levels [43–53]. In addition to triggering genes (with progesterone) that are crucial for implantation and placentation, IFN-τ, as a key regulator of the immune response of the pregnant cow, has immunomodulatory influence on several types of cells, including neutrophils, and antiproliferative, antiluteolytic, and immunosuppressive effects on the endometrium [43–55].

How Does the Immune System Aid in Maintaining Pregnancy?

Once an implantation has occurred, the maternal–fetal interface, called the placenta, develops [56]. Even though the placenta serves as an anatomical barrier between fetus and mother (with separate circulatory systems), the placenta is abundant with immune cells and mediators. These cells not only protect the fetus from infections but also aid in fetal development and prevent immune responses aimed at the fetus [8, 57–59]. These cells include the following:

A. Monocytes and macrophages are recruited to the pregnant endometrium in cattle [76], while not all of their functions are known, known functions include clearing of apoptotic cells, regulation of apoptosis, curtailing the activation of anticonceptus immune responses, and regulation of placental lactogen levels [8, 58–64]. These cells are essential for maintaining pregnancy [64].
B. Immature dendritic cells are in high numbers in the endometria of cows and may be involved with the induction and maintenance of immune tolerance in response to IFN-τ [65, 66].
C. Lymphocytes (particularly T-lymphocytes) are critical for maintaining the pregnancy once IFN-τ release is completed. Regulatory T-cells (Tregs) mediate maternal-fetal tolerance. This includes effector T-cell regulation, interactions with innate immune cells in the uterine microenvironment, and modulation of trophoblast function [2, 8, 67, 68].

The presence of the bovine fetus stimulates the cellular expansion of T cells (CD4+, CD8+, γδ+) and B cell populations in the endometrium [59, 69, 70]. There is, however, a modulation of the cytokine and mRNA expressed by these cells, altering their function during pregnancy [71, 72].

Another unique feature of ruminant pregnancy (in addition to IFN-τ) is the small role natural killer (NK) cells play during pregnancy. In other species (mouse and human), NK cells comprise most of the endometrial lymphocytes and are a significant contributor to pregnancy in those species [8, 66, 73].

As pregnancy progresses, the immune system changes to protect both mother and fetus. Bovine maternal immunity changes from type 1 (cell-mediated response) to predominantly type 2 (antibody-mediated immune response) during pregnancy [74]. If this shift does not occur, pregnancy is not maintained. This drives the immune system towards a more anti-inflammatory state, preventing the rejection of the developing fetus during gestation [8, 43, 74–76]. There is an increase in circulating levels of anti-inflammatory cytokines and chemokines, such as IL-10 and TGF-β. This also corresponds to an increase in the number of Tregs in the maternal circulation and suppressed activity of cells that could target the fetus, such as cytotoxic T cells [43, 74–76]. The shift from Th1 to Th2 response as pregnancy progresses protects the mother and the fetus and prepares for the movement of antibodies to the udder as colostrum forms.

Beginning at approximately 3 weeks prior to calving, systemic immunosuppression occurs in the pregnant ruminant. Immunologic dysfunction of both lymphocytes and neutrophils has been demonstrated [77–83]. While increased immune suppression can be measured beginning 3 weeks prepartum, broad systemic immune suppression is more dramatic in the first 2 weeks postpartum [77–83]. The exact causes of immune suppression in these animals are not clear; hormonal and metabolic changes are thought to influence the suppression of the systemic immune response [84, 85].

While the systemic immune system is undergoing suppression, late pregnancy and parturition do not have the same effect on the mucosal immune system [86, 87]. Some of the decrease in systemic immune cells attributed to calving immune suppression may be shifting from the systemic immune system to the uterus. There is an influx of neutrophils into the uterus, and uterine lymphocytes, eosinophils, mast cells, and macrophages are activated [84, 88–95]. Neutrophils play a primary role in the defense of the uterus against infection and are critical for the expulsion of the *placenta* [84, 88–95].

The major classes of immunoglobulins (IgM, IgA, and IgG) assist in antibacterial defenses via opsonization, complement activation, and/or neutralization of pathogens and may be locally produced or moved from the systemic immune system. Further movement of systemic immune components to the local immune system occurs with the formation of colostrum (see Chap. 7) [96, 97].

Conclusion

While the impact of hormones, genomics, and nutrition on bovine reproduction is well understood, the influence of the immune system is still an area of discovery. All aspects of reproduction have immunologic inputs and controls. As more information is uncovered, new methods for impacting infertility and pregnancy loss may be found.

Your Case

History

200 cow Registered Holstein dairy in the Midwest. Cattle are housed in free stall barns and fed a total mixed ration, corn silage, and alfalfa hay. Calves are raised on site. A nutritionist manages the ration. Vaccination program of the cows includes: Modified live virus vaccine containing Bovine viral diarrhea virus (type 1 and 2), Bovine herpesvirus 1, Parainfluenza 3, and Bovine respiratory syncytial virus, and inactivated *Leptospira canicola, grippotyphosa, Hardjo-bovis icterohaemorrhagiae,* and *pomona* bacterin (five-way) at 35 days in milk. At pregnancy confirmation (60 days of pregnancy), a second five-way Leptospira vaccination is administered. At cessation of milking (dry off-60 days pre-calving) and 30 days pre-calving, a core *E.coli* bacterin is administered (J5). Cows calve in calving pens and are moved to post-calving (fresh) pens (free stalls), where they remain for 35 days, when they are moved into the lactating pens (free stalls). The herd has a 305-day RHA of 26,300 pounds, with three times a day milking.

Reproductive Management

Cows are palpated at 14–21 days post-calving for normal uterine involution. Ultrasound pregnancy checks are performed at approximately 30 days post-breeding, and the pregnancy is ultrasound confirmed at 60–75 days of pregnancy. The herd utilizes a timed AI program with a 45-day voluntary waiting period. The herd is semi-closed with an occasional pregnant heifer being added.

Problem

Beginning 36 months ago, the herd began to experience a precipitous drop in reproductive efficiency as follows:

Services per conception 2.0–3.1
First service conception rate 45% to 37%
Early embryonic fetal loss 9.6–19%
Annual reproductive cull rate 7–18%
Estrus cycle also increased to an average of 29 days

It should be noted that genomic selection for reproductive traits was not available at the time of this case.

Questions

1. Where do you start to work up this complex problem?
2. Based on initial diagnostics, what do you recommend?
3. What results do you anticipate within 6 months of the program?
4. If unsatisfactory results after 6 months, what further diagnostics would you run?
5. Based on further testing, what changes would you make to the program?

Additional Readings

1. Diskin MG, Morris DG. Embryonic and early foetal losses in cattle and other ruminants. Reprod Domest Anim. 2008;43(Suppl 2):260–7. https://doi.org/10.1111/j.1439-0531.2008.01171.x. PMID: 18638133.
2. Pandit A, Shah SM, Shah RA, Qureshi S, Sethi RS, Bhat F, Malik A, Parray O, Yaqoob H, Saleem M. Regulatory T cells in bovine fertility: Current understanding and future prospects. Anim Reprod Sci. 2025;272:107655. ISSN 0378-4320. https://doi.org/10.1016/j.anireprosci.2024.107655.
3. LeBlanc SJ. Postpartum uterine disease and dairy herd reproductive performance: a review. Vet J. 2008;176(1):102–14. https://doi.org/10.1016/j.tvjl.2007.12.019. Epub 2008 Mar 6. PMID: 18328749.
4. Deori S, Phookan A. Bovine postpartum metritis and its therapeutics: a review. Indian J Sci Technol. 2015;8:1–5. https://doi.org/10.17485/ijst/2015/v8i23/52386.
5. Lamb GC, Mercadante VR. Synchronization and artificial insemination strategies in beef cattle. Vet Clin North Am Food Anim Pract. 2016;32(2):335–47. https://doi.org/10.1016/j.cvfa.2016.01.006.
6. Medawar P. Some immunological and endocrinological problems raised by the evolution of viviparity in vertebrates. Symp Soc Exp Biol. 1953;7:320–38.
7. Petroff MG, Nguyen SL, Ahn SH. Fetal-placental antigens and the maternal immune system: reproductive immunology comes of age. Immunol Rev. 2022;308(1):25–39. https://doi.org/10.1111/imr.13090. Epub 2022 May 29. PMID: 35643905; PMCID: PMC9328203.
8. Fair T. The contribution of the maternal immune system to the establishment of pregnancy in cattle. Front Immunol. 2015;6:7. https://doi.org/10.3389/fimmu.2015.00007. PMID: 25674085; PMCID: PMC4309202. D: 11692509.
9. Hunter AG. Immunology and fertility in the bovine. J Dairy Sci. 1989;72(12):3353–62. ISSN 0022-0302,. https://doi.org/10.3168/jds.S0022-0302(89)79498-4.
10. Webb R, Armstrong DG. Control of ovarian function; effect of local interactions and environmental influences on follicular turnover in cattle: a review. Livest Prod Sci. 1998;53(2):95–112. ISSN 0301-6226. https://doi.org/10.1016/S0301-6226(97)00161-9.
11. Alrabiah N, Evans A, Fahey A, Cantwell N, Lonergan P, McCormack J, Browne J, Fair T. Immunological aspects of follicle ovulation and corpus luteum formation in cattle. Reproduction. 2021;162:209–25. https://doi.org/10.1530/REP-21-0165.
12. Ye H, Li X, Zheng T, Liang X, Li J, Huang J, Pan Z, Zhen Y. The effect of the immune system on ovarian function and features of ovarian germline stem cells. Springerplus. 2016;5:990. https://doi.org/10.1186/s40064-016-2390-3.
13. Crespo D, Bonnet E, Roher N, MacKenzie SA, Krasnov A, Goetz FW, Bobe J, Planas JV. Cellular and molecular evidence for a role of tumor necrosis factor alpha in the ovulatory mechanism of trout. Reprod Biol Endocrinol. 2010;8(34).
14. Cacciottola L, Camboni A, Dolmans MM. Immune system regulation of physiological and pathological aspects of the ovarian follicle pool throughout the female reproductive lifespan. Hum Reprod. 2025;40(1):12–22. https://doi.org/10.1093/humrep/deae254. PMID: 39607771.

15. Herath S, Williams EJ, Lilly ST, Gilbert RO, Dobson H, Bryant CE, Sheldon IM. Ovarian follicular cells have innate immune capabilities that modulate their endocrine function. Reproduction. 2007;134(5):683–93. https://doi.org/10.1530/REP-07-0229. PMID: 17965259; PMCID: PMC2735812.
16. Li J, Zhou F, Zheng T, et al. Ovarian germline stem cells (OGSCs) and the hippo signaling pathway association with physiological and pathological ovarian aging in mice. Cell Physiol Biochem. 2015;36(5):1712–24. https://doi.org/10.1159/000430144.
17. Bukovsky A. Ovarian stem cell niche and follicular renewal in mammals. Anat Rec. 2011;294(8):1284–306. https://doi.org/10.1002/ar.21422.
18. Nakao K, Kishi H, Imai F, Suwa H, Hirakawa T, Minegishi T. TNF-alpha suppressed FSH-induced LH receptor expression through transcriptional regulation in rat granulosa cells. Endocrinology. 2015;156(9):3192–202. https://doi.org/10.1210/EN.2015-1238.
19. Gerard N, Caillaud M, Martoriati A, Goudet G, Lalmanach AC. The interleukin-1 system and female reproduction. J Endocrinol. 2004;180(2):203–12. https://doi.org/10.1677/joe.0.1800203.
20. Galvao AM, Ferreira-Dias G, Skarzynski DJ. Cytokines and angiogenesis in the corpus luteum. Mediators Inflamm. 2013;2013:420186. https://doi.org/10.1155/2013/420186.
21. Galvão AM, Szóstek AZ, Skarzynski DJ, Ferreira-Dias GM. Role of tumor necrosis factor-α, interferon-γ and Fas-ligand on in vitro nitric oxide activity in the corpus luteum. Cytokine. 2013;64(1):18–21. https://doi.org/10.1016/j.cyto.2013.07.015.
22. Fedorcsák P, Polec A, Ráki M, Holm R, Jebsen P, Åbyholm T. Differential release of matrix metalloproteinases and tissue inhibitors of metalloproteinases by human granulosa-lutein cells and ovarian leukocytes. Endocrinology. 2010;151(3):1290–8. https://doi.org/10.1210/en.2009-0605.
23. Penny LA, Armstrong D, Bramley TA, Webb R, Collins RA, Watson ED. Immune cells and cytokine production in the bovine corpus luteum throughout the oestrous cycle and after induced luteolysis. J Reprod Fertil. 1999;115(1):87–96. https://doi.org/10.1530/jrf.0.1150087.
24. Bauer M, Reibiger I, Spanel-Borowski K. Leucocyte proliferation in the bovine corpus luteum. Reproduction. 2001;121(2):297–305. https://doi.org/10.1530/rep.0.1210297.
25. Poole DH, Pate JL. Luteal microenvironment directs resident T lymphocyte function in cows. Biol Reprod. 2012;86(2):29. https://doi.org/10.1095/biolreprod.111.092296.
26. Pandya IJ, Cohen J. The leukocytic reaction of the human uterine cervix to spermatozoa. Fertil Steril. 1985;43(3):417–21.
27. Robertson SA. Seminal plasma and male factor signalling in the female reproductive tract. Cell Tissue Res. 2005;322(1):43–52. https://doi.org/10.1007/s00441-005-1127-3.
28. Robertson SA, Mau VJ, Tremellen KP, Seamark RF. Role of high molecular weight seminal vesicle proteins in eliciting the uterine inflammatory response to semen in mice. J Reprod Fertil. 1996;107(2):265–77. https://doi.org/10.1530/jrf.0.1070265.
29. Sharkey DJ, Macpherson AM, Tremellen KP, Mottershead DG, Gilchrist RB, Robertson SA. TGF-beta mediates proinflammatory seminal fluid signaling in human cervical epithelial cells. J Immunol. 2012;189(2):1024–35. https://doi.org/10.4049/jimmunol.1200005.
30. Rubtsov YP, Rudensky AY. TGFbeta signalling in control of T-cell-mediated self-reactivity. Nat Rev Immunol. 2007;7(6):443–53. https://doi.org/10.1038/nri2095.
31. Tremellen KP, Seamark RF, Robertson SA. Seminal transforming growth factor beta1 stimulates granulocyte-macrophage colony-stimulating factor production and inflammatory cell recruitment in the murine uterus. Biol Reprod. 1998;58(5):1217–25. https://doi.org/10.1095/biolreprod58.5.1217.
32. Mattner PE. The distribution of spermatozoa and leucocytes in the female genital tract in goats and cattle. J Reprod Fertil. 1968;17(2):253–61. https://doi.org/10.1530/jrf.0.0170253.
33. Tomlinson MJ, White A, Barratt CL, Bolton AE, Cooke ID. The removal of morphologically abnormal sperm forms by phagocytes: a positive role for seminal leukocytes? Hum Reprod. 1992;7(4):517–22.
34. Troedsson MH, Liu IK, Crabo BG. Sperm transport and survival in the mare. Theriogenology. 1998;49(5):905–15. https://doi.org/10.1016/S0093-691X(98)00040-5.

35. Moldenhauer LM, Diener KR, Thring DM, Brown MP, Hayball JD, Robertson SA. Cross-presentation of male seminal fluid antigens elicits T cell activation to initiate the female immune response to pregnancy. J Immunol. 2009;182(12):8080–93. https://doi.org/10.4049/jimmunol.0804018.
36. Waberski D, Dohring A, Ardon F, Ritter N, Zerbe H, Schuberth HJ, et al. Physiological routes from intra-uterine seminal contents to advancement of ovulation. Acta Vet Scand. 2006;48:13. https://doi.org/10.1186/1751-0147-48-S1-S13.
37. Odhiambo JF, Poole DH, Hughes L, Dejarnette JM, Inskeep EK, Dailey RA. Pregnancy outcome in dairy and beef cattle after artificial insemination and treatment with seminal plasma or transforming growth factor beta-1. Theriogenology. 2009;72(4):566–71. https://doi.org/10.1016/j.theriogenology.2009.04.013.
38. Lima FS, Risco CA, Thatcher MJ, Benzaquen ME, Archbald LF, Santos JE, et al. Comparison of reproductive performance in lactating dairy cows bred by natural service or timed artificial insemination. J Dairy Sci. 2009;92(11):5456–66. https://doi.org/10.3168/jds.2009-2197.
39. Robertson SA, Guerin LR, Moldenhauer LM, Hayball JD. Activating T regulatory cells for tolerance in early pregnancy—the contribution of seminal fluid. J Reprod Immunol. 2009;83(1–2):109–16. https://doi.org/10.1016/j.jri.2009.08.003. [DOI] [PubMed] [Google Scholar].
40. Spencer TE, Johnson GA, Bazer FW, Burghardt RC, Palmarini M. Pregnancy recognition and conceptus implantation in domestic ruminants: roles of progesterone, interferons and endogenous retroviruses. Reprod Fertil Dev. 2007;19(1):65–78. https://doi.org/10.1071/RD06102.
41. Lin H, Mosmann TR, Guilbert L, Tuntipopipat S, Wegmann TG. Synthesis of T helper 2-type cytokines at the maternal-fetal interface. J Immunol. 1993;151(9):4562–73.
42. Chaouat G. The Th1/Th2 paradigm: still important in pregnancy? Semin Immunopathol. 2007;29(2):95–113. https://doi.org/10.1007/s00281-007-0069-0.
43. Mor G, Cardenas I. The immune system in pregnancy: a unique complexity. Am J Reprod Immunol. 2010;63(6):425–33. https://doi.org/10.1111/j.1600-0897.2010.00836.x. Epub 2010 Mar 29. PMID: 20367629; PMCID: PMC3025805.
44. Manjari P, Hyder I, Kapoor S, Senthilnathan M, Dang AK. Exploring the concentration-dependent actions of interferon-τ on bovine neutrophils to understand the process of implantation. J Cell Biochem. 2018;119(12):10087–94. https://doi.org/10.1002/jcb.27345. PMID 30171720. S2CID 206028552.
45. Shirasuna K, Matsumoto H, Matsuyama S, Kimura K, Bollwein H, Miyamoto A. Possible role of interferon tau on the bovine corpus luteum and neutrophils during the early pregnancy. Reproduction. 2015;150(3):217–25. https://doi.org/10.1530/REP-15-0085. PMID 26078085.
46. Racicot K, Kwon JY, Aldo P, Silasi M, Mor G. Understanding the complexity of the immune system during pregnancy. Am J Reprod Immunol. 2014;72(2):107–16. https://doi.org/10.1111/aji.12289. Epub 2014 Jul 4. PMID: 24995526; PMCID: PMC6800182.
47. Brooks K, Spencer TE. Biological roles of interferon tau (IFNT) and type I IFN receptors in elongation of the ovine conceptus. Biol Reprod. 2015;92(2):47. https://doi.org/10.1095/biolreprod.114.124156. PMID 25505203.
48. Spencer TE, Ott TL, Bazer FW. Expression of interferon regulatory factors one and two in the ovine endometrium: effects of pregnancy and ovine interferon tau. Biol Reprod. 1998;58(5):1154–62. https://doi.org/10.1095/biolreprod58.5.1154. PMID 9603248.
49. Stewart MD, Stewart DM, Johnson GA, Vyhlidal CA, Burghardt RC, Safe SH, Yu-Lee LY, Bazer FW, Spencer TE. Interferon-tau activates multiple signal transducer and activator of transcription proteins and has complex effects on interferon-responsive gene transcription in ovine endometrial epithelial cells. Endocrinology. 2001;142(1):98–107. https://doi.org/10.1210/endo.142.1.7891. PMID 11145571.
50. Platanias LC. Mechanisms of type-I- and type-II-interferon-mediated signalling. Nat Rev Immunol. 2005;5(5):375–86. https://doi.org/10.1038/nri1604. PMID 15864272.
51. Tanikawa N, Seno K, Kawahara-Miki R, Kimura K, Matsuyama S, Iwata H, Kuwayama T, Shirasuna K. Interferon tau regulates cytokine production and cellular function in human

trophoblast cell line. J Interf Cytokine Res. 2017;37(10):456–66. https://doi.org/10.1089/jir.2017.0057. PMID 29028431.
52. Hansen TR, Sinedino LD, Spencer TE. Paracrine and endocrine actions of interferon tau (IFNT). Reproduction. 2017;154(5):F45–59. https://doi.org/10.1530/REP-17-0315. PMID 28982937.
53. Bazer FW, Thatcher WW. Chronicling the discovery of interferon taa. Reproduction. 2017;154(5):F11–20. https://doi.org/10.1530/REP-17-0257. PMC 5630494. PMID 28747540.
54. Ott TL, Fleming JG, Spencer TE, Joyce MM, Chen P, Green CN, Zhu D, Welsh TH Jr, Harms PG, Bazer FW. Effects of exogenous recombinant ovine interferon tau on circulating concentrations of progesterone, cortisol, luteinizing hormone, and antiviral activity; interestrous interval; rectal temperature; and uterine response to oxytocin in cyclic ewes. Biol Reprod. 1997;57(3):621–9. https://doi.org/10.1095/biolreprod57.3.621.
55. Choi Y, Johnson GA, Spencer TE, Bazer FW. Pregnancy and interferon tau regulate major histocompatibility complex class I and beta2-microglobulin expression in the ovine uterus. Biol Reprod. 2003;68(5):1703–10. https://doi.org/10.1095/biolreprod.102.012708.
56. Schlafer DH, Fisher PJ, Davies CJ. The bovine placenta before and after birth: placental development and function in health and disease. Anim Reprod Sci. 2000;60-61:145–60. https://doi.org/10.1016/s0378-4320(00)00132-9.
57. Wegmann TG. Maternal T cells promote placental growth and prevent spontaneous abortion. Immunol Lett. 1988;17(4):297–302. https://doi.org/10.1016/0165-2478(88)90001-6.
58. Oliveira L, Barreto R, Perecin F, Mansouri-Attia N, Pereira F, Meirelles F. Modulation of maternal immune system during pregnancy in the cow. Reprod Domest Anim. 2012;47:384–93. https://doi.org/10.1111/j.1439-0531.2012.02102.x.
59. Rutigliano HM, Leppo KA, Morgado KP. Changes in mononuclear immune cells during bovine pregnancy. Reprod Fertil Dev. 2021;34(8):608–18. https://doi.org/10.1071/RD21161.
60. Oliveira LJ, McClellan S, Hansen PJ. Differentiation of the endometrial macrophage during pregnancy in the cow. PLoS One. 2010;5(10):e13213. https://doi.org/10.1371/journal.pone.0013213.
61. Oliveira LJ, Hansen PJ. Phenotypic characterization of macrophages in the endometrium of the pregnant cow. Am J Reprod Immunol. 2009;62(6):418–26. https://doi.org/10.1111/j.1600-0897.2009.00761.x.
62. Straszewski-Chavez SL, Abrahams VM, Mor G. The role of apoptosis in the regulation of trophoblast survival and differentiation during pregnancy. Endocr Rev. 2005;26(7):877–97. https://doi.org/10.1210/er.2005-0003.
63. Kzhyshkowska J, Gratchev A, Schmuttermaier C, Brundiers H, Krusell L, Mamidi S, et al. Alternatively activated macrophages regulate extracellular levels of the hormone placental lactogen via receptor-mediated uptake and transcytosis. J Immunol. 2008;180(5):3028–37. https://doi.org/10.4049/jimmunol.180.5.3028.
64. Wang LL, Li ZH, Wang H, Kwak-Kim J, Liao AH. Cutting edge: the regulatory mechanisms of macrophage polarization and function during pregnancy. J Reprod Immunol. 2022;151:103627. ISSN 0165-0378. https://doi.org/10.1016/j.jri.2022.103627.
65. Mansouri-Attia N, Oliveira LJ, Forde N, Fahey AG, Browne JA, Roche JF, Sandra O, Reinaud P, Lonergan P, Fair T. Pivotal role for monocytes/macrophages and dendritic cells in maternal immune response to the developing embryo in cattle. Biol Reprod. 2012;87(5):123. https://doi.org/10.1095/biolreprod.112.101121.
66. Dietl J, Honig A, Kammerer U, Rieger L. Natural killer cells and dendritic cells at the human feto-maternal interface: an effective cooperation? Placenta. 2006;27(4–5):341–7. https://doi.org/10.1016/j.placenta.2005.05.001.
67. Huang N, Chi H, Qiao J. Role of regulatory T cells in regulating fetal-maternal immune tolerance in healthy pregnancies and reproductive diseases. Front Immunol. 2020;11:1023. https://doi.org/10.3389/fimmu.2020.01023. PMID: 32676072; PMCID: PMC7333773.
68. Maeda Y, Ohtsuka H, Tomioka M, Oikawa M. Effect of progesterone on Th1/Th2/Th17 and regulatory T cell-related genes in peripheral blood mononuclear cells during pregnancy in cows. Vet Res Commun. 2013;37(1):43–9. https://doi.org/10.1007/s11259-012-9545-7.

69. Cobb SP, Watson ED. Immunohistochemical study of immune cells in the bovine endometrium at different stages of the oestrous cycle. Res Vet Sci. 1995;59:238–41. https://doi.org/10.1016/0034-5288(95)90010-1.
70. Dimova T, Mihaylova A, Fettke F, Schumacher A, Costa S-D, Zenclussen AC. B cells: the old new players in reproductive immunology. Front Immunol. 2014;5:285. https://doi.org/10.3389/fimmu.2014.00285.
71. Kamat MM, Vasudevan S, Maalouf SA, Townson DH, Pate JL, Ott TL. Changes in myeloid lineage cells in the uterus and peripheral blood of dairy heifers during early pregnancy. Biol Reprod. 2016;95:68. https://doi.org/10.1095/biolreprod.116.141069617.
72. Vasudevan S, Kamat MM, Walusimbi SS, Pate JL, Ott TL. Effects of early pregnancy on uterine lymphocytes and endometrial expression of immune-regulatory molecules in dairy heifers. Biol Reprod. 2017;97:104–18. https://doi.org/10.1093/biolre/iox061.
73. Oliveira LJ, Mansourri-Attia N, Fahey AG, Browne J, Forde N, Roche JF, PatLonergan P, Trudee Fair T. Characterization of the Th profile of the bovine endometrium during the oestrous cycle and early pregnancy. PLoS One. 2013;8(10):e75571. https://doi.org/10.1371/journal.pone.0075571.
74. Abu-Raya B, Michalski C, Sadarangani M, Lavoie PM. Maternal immunological adaptation during normal pregnancy. Front Immunol. 2020;11:575197. https://doi.org/10.3389/fimmu.2020.575197. PMID: 33133091; PMCID: PMC7579415.
75. Corpron M, Ahmadzadeh A, Rezamand P, Huo Q. Relationship between beef cow fertility and maternal immunity. Appl. Anim Sci. 2021;37(6):733–7. ISSN 2590-2865. https://doi.org/10.15232/aas.2021-02214.
76. Orefice R. Immunology and the immunological response in pregnancy. Best Pract Res Clin Obstet Gynaecol. 2021;76:3–12. https://doi.org/10.1016/j.bpobgyn.2020.07.013. Epub 2020 Oct 14. PMID: 33191116.
77. Aleri JW, Hine BC, Pyman, Mansell PD, Wales WJ, Mallard B, Fisher AD. Periparturient immunosuppression and strategies to improve dairy cow health during the periparturient period. Res Vet Sci. 2016;108:8–17. ISSN 0034-5288. https://doi.org/10.1016/j.rvsc.2016.07.007.
78. Burton JL, Madsen SA, Chang LC, Weber PS, Buckham KR, van Dorp R, Hickey MC, Earley B. Gene expression signatures in neutrophils exposed to glucocorticoids: a new paradigm to help explain "neutrophil dysfunction" in parturient dairy cows. Vet Immunol Immunopathol. 2005;105:197–219.
79. Comline RS, Hall LW, Lavelle RB, Nathanielsz PW, Silverg M. Parturition in the cow: endocrine changes in animals with chronically implanted catheters in the foetal and maternal circulations. J Endocrinol. 1974;63:451–72.
80. Detilleux JC, Kehrli ME Jr, Stabel JR, Freeman AE, Kelley DH. Study of immunological dysfunction in periparturient Holstein cattle selected for high and average milk production. Vet Immunol Immunopathol. 1995;44(3):251–67.
81. Kehrli ME Jr, Nonnecke BJ, Roth JA. Alterations in bovine neutrophil function during the periparturient period. Am J Vet Res. 1986;50:207–14.
82. Kehrli ME Jr, Nonnecke BJ, Roth JA. Alterations in bovine lymphocyte function during the periparturient period. Am J Vet Res. 1989;50(2):215–20.
83. Ishikawa H, Shirahata T, Hasegawa K. Interferon-γ production of mitogen stimulated peripheral lymphocytes in perinatal cows. J Vet Med Sci. 1994;56(4):735–8.
84. Kimura K, Goff JP, Kehrli ME Jr, Reinhardt TA. Decreased neutrophil function as a cause of retained placenta in dairy cattle. J Dairy Sci. 2002;85(3):544–50.
85. Kimura K, Goff JP, Kehrli ME, et al. J Dairy Sci. 1999;82:2385–92.
86. Cortese VS, Woolums A, Hurley DJ, Berghaus R, Bernard JK, Short TH. Comparison of interferon and bovine herpesvirus-1-specific IgA levels in nasal secretions of dairy cattle administered an intranasal modified live viral vaccine prior to calving or on the day of calving. Vet Immunol Immunopathol. 2017;187:35–41.
87. Cortese VS, Woolums A, Thoresen M, Pinedo PJ, Short T. Mucosal immune responses in peri-parturient dairy cattle. Vet Microbiol. 2024;298:110201. ISSN 0378-1135. https://doi.org/10.1016/j.vetmic.2024.110201.

88. Singh J, Murray RD, Mshelia G, Woldehiwet Z. The immune status of the bovine uterus during the peripartum period. Vet J. 2008;175(3):301–9. ISSN 1090-0233. https://doi.org/10.1016/j.tvjl.2007.02.003.
89. Gunnink JW. Post-partum leucocytic activity and its relationship to caesarian section and retained placenta. Vet Q. 1984;6:55–7.
90. Gunnink JW. Pre-partum leucotytic activity and retained placenta. Vet Q. 1984;6:52–4.
91. Gunnink JW. Retained placenta and leukocytic activity. Vet Q. 1984;6:49–51.
92. Heuwieser W, Grunert E. Significance of chemotactic activity for placental expulsion in cattle. Theriogenology. 1987;27:907–12.
93. Hoedemaker M, Lund LA, Wagner WC. Function of neutrophils and chemoattractant properties of fetal placenta tissue during the last month of pregnancy in cows. Am J Vet Res. 1992;53:1524–9.
94. Cai T-Q, Weston PG, Lund LA, Brodie B, McKenna DJ, Wagner WC. Association between neutrophil functions and periparturient disorders in cows. Am J Vet Res. 1994;55:934–43.
95. Romaniukowa K. Phagocytosis in the uterus. In: Proceedings of the 10th international congress animal reproduction artificial insemination. Champaign-Urbana: University of Illinois; 1994. p. 33–8.
96. Stelwagen K, Carpenter E, Haigh B, Hodgkinson A, Wheeler TT. Immune components of bovine colostrum and milk. J Anim Sci. 2009;87(13 Suppl):3–9. https://doi.org/10.2527/jas.2008-1377.
97. Playford RJ, Weiser MJ. Bovine colostrum: its constituents and uses. Nutrients. 2021;13(1):265. https://doi.org/10.3390/nu13010265. PMID: 33477653; PMCID: PMC7831509.
98. Cortese VS, Behan S, Galvin JE, Penka DR, Ramsey D, Bryson WL, Lucas MJ. Evaluation of two antimicrobial therapies in the treatment of Leptospira borgpetersenii serovar hardjo infection in experimentally infected cattle. Vet Ther. 2007;8(3):201–8. PMID: 17926305.

Mammary Gland Immunity During Infection (Mastitis)

11

Abstract

Globally, *mastitis* is still the costliest disease to the dairy industry. Losses include decreased milk production, discarded milk, treatment costs, and cows culled due to chronic mastitis. While a few infections can occur from a systemic infection, most mastitis arises from pathogens ascending the teat canal. The barrier defenses of the teat canal are part of the local immune system; however, the systemic immune system is involved in responses to infections within the mammary gland. The goal of the immune response in the infected quarter is twofold: to minimize inflammation and to remove the pathogen.

Keywords

Mastitis · mammary gland · coliform mastitis · *Escherichia coli* · *Staphylococcus aureus* · endotoxin

Key Concepts

- Mastitis is defined as inflammation of the mammary gland. In cattle, it is typically caused by an infection.
- Most infections enter through the teat canal when barrier defenses are disrupted or inadequate.
- Immune responses target microbial invader(s) in order to reduce inflammation and minimize or prevent permanent gland damage.
- Some organisms that evade the immune response or escape veterinary medical intervention can cause severe disease, ranging from permanent damage to the mammary gland tissues and death.

J. Ellis, V. Cortese, *Practical Bovine Immunology*,
https://doi.org/10.1007/978-3-032-15031-8_11

What Is Mastitis?

Bovine mastitis is defined as *inflammation* within the mammary gland [1]. Most mastitis cases are due to bacterial, fungal, viral, or algal infections of the mammary gland, although not all mastitis is caused by an infection and can be observed with physical trauma to the mammary gland. Seen in all species of lactating mammals, it is most commonly seen in animals used for dairy production [1–3]. Mastitis is a major cause of economic loss in the dairy industry worldwide and is most often categorized into clinical and subclinical mastitis [4, 5]. The inflammation can be caused by an extensive list of microbes, including *Pasteurella multocida, Staphylococcus aureus, Streptococcus (Str.) zooepidemicus, Str. agalactiae, Str. pyogenes, Str. faecalis, Mycobacterium bovis, Klebsiella* spp., *Brucella abortus, Pseudomonas pyocyaneus, E. coli,* and *Leptospira Pomona.* Cows with *clinical mastitis* have visible signs of mastitis, including abnormal milk and swelling of an infected quarter. Milk from a mammary gland with mastitis may contain blood or milk clots and appear discolored and have a fetid odor. Cows suffering from clinical mastitis may have poor appetites and other clinical signs of discomfort, including stiffened gait due to swollen udders, diarrhea, and evidence of dehydration. Fever, anorexia, and dehydration can be seen in severe cases, and death can occur. Cows with *subclinical mastitis* display no apparent signs of the disease but will have increased somatic cells (detected by various methods, i.e., the California Mastitis Test) in the milk and often are culture positive for bacteria.

What Happens as Pathogens Get Past the Teat Canal Barrier?

As pointed out in Chap. 6, *the teat canal barrier* maintains the aseptic nature of the mammary gland [3, 6, 7]. An inflammatory response is initiated when a pathogen invades the mammary gland or tissue injury occurs with the goal of restoring immune homeostasis, removing the invader, and returning the affected quarter to normal function. If the immune response is too slow, not strong enough, or dysfunctional, severe acute inflammation or chronic mastitis may occur [8].

Is the Immune Response the Same for All Causes of Mastitis?

The effectiveness of the mammary gland immune system determines the ability of cows to resist the establishment of new intramammary infections. While there are some immune responses that are specific to a particular pathogen, the general immune responses are similar whenever mammary gland damage occurs.

As with other immunological systems in the body, the mammary immune system comprises innate and adaptive immune responses. The innate immune system responds very quickly to pathogen invasion and begins with the epithelial cells of the teat duct. These cells can express pathogen recognition receptors and Toll-like receptors (TLRs) that bind to pathogen-associated molecular patterns. Cytokines (interleukin (IL)-1beta, tumor necrosis factor (TNF)-alpha, IL-8), acute phase proteins (haptoglobin), and antimicrobial peptides (pentraxin 3 and lipopolysaccharide-binding protein) are released, and inflammatory genes are expressed [9, 10]. Similar actions can occur in the mammary gland as well. Both upregulated neutrophils and macrophages then respond and engage in phagocytosis. As with other immunological systems, mammary macrophages function as antigen-presenting cells [11, 12]. IL-2, in conjunction with antigen presentation, regulates the bovine mammary gland adaptive immune system, stimulating B lymphocyte proliferation, improving the effectiveness of T lymphocytes, increasing plasma cell numbers, and activating natural killer (NK) cells [10, 13–15].

While the adaptive immune response in the udder may take several days to develop, the response is more specific to select factors that cause mastitis. *The mammary gland* of dairy cattle contains the full repertoire of lymphocytes (Th1, Th2, Th17, Treg, T cytotoxic, gamma-delta T cells, and B cells), but the number of each subset of lymphocytes varies by stage of lactation [3, 16–18]. CD4+ cells are the predominant activated cells during mastitis and drive immune responses by other lymphocytes via cytokine release (CD8+ and gamma delta T cells) [17, 18]. As macrophages, neutrophils, and lymphocytes move into the mammary gland, there is a corresponding increase in somatic cell counts in milk. Three important cytokines, IL-4, IL-10, and IL-17A, are released by CD4+ Th2 cells (as well as other cells) during mastitis events. IL-4 is one of the most important B cell activation cytokines; IL-4 drives antibody responses, stimulating B cells to grow and differentiate into active plasma cells or memory cells [19–22]. This may be an indication of the importance of antibodies in providing protection against and clearance of many mastitis-causing agents.

IL-10 plays a major role in protecting and healing the mammary mucosa from damage. This cytokine functions as an anti-inflammatory cytokine by suppressing different immune cells (CD4+ and CD8+ T cells, B cells, antigen-presenting cells, NK cells, and macrophages) and pro-inflammatory cytokines (IL-6, IL-8, and TNF-α) [19–21].

IL-17A is a pro-inflammatory cytokine, and production of IL-17A is induced during clinical and subclinical mastitis by several different mastitis-causing agents. Similar to IL-4, IL-17A is involved in the initiation of antigen-specific mammary inflammation by increasing phagocytosis and antigen presentation as well as the activation of epithelial cells, fibroblasts, and endothelial cells [19–21].

Tregs release transforming growth factor-beta 1 (TGF-β1), which is another anti-inflammatory cytokine. With IL-10, TGFβ-1 suppresses macrophages and other immune cells (CD4+ and CD8+ T cells, B cells, antigen-presenting cells, and NK cells) and different pro-inflammatory factors' activity, and protects and aids in healing mammary mucosa [19]. The immune response to mastitis is a complex immunologic interaction aimed at clearing the invader while simultaneously minimizing damage to the organ. This shows that the primary immune response against mastitis is phagocytic, humoral, and cytokine/chemokine mediated. The action of CD8+ and gamma delta cells in mastitis is unclear.

Two notable exceptions to the general immune responses listed above are as follows:

A. Mastitis caused by *Gram-negative coliforms* can range from subclinical to severe peracute to acute cases with sepsis and systemic endotoxic involvement that can often lead to death. While *E. coli* is the most common cause of coliform mastitis, it can also be caused by *Klebsiella* species [23–27]. Clinical coliform mastitis cases are associated with a fast and dramatic immune response with pro-inflammatory cytokines released and severe inflammation in the infected quarter, which can activate the TLR4 signaling pathway in bovine mammary epithelial cells [24]. TLR4 interacts with LPS components of the cell walls of Gram-negative bacteria, thereby triggering the activation of NF-κB and mitogen-activated protein kinase signaling pathways. Bacterial sepsis and septic and endotoxic shock result from the overproduction of inflammatory mediators from the interaction of the immune system with lipopolysaccharides (endotoxin) and other bacterial cell wall constituents in the body. While the immune responses listed above are important for the prevention and control of coliform mastitis, the speed of the pathogenesis and systemic involvement are often faster than the immune system response [27, 28]. The use of endotoxin core mutant vaccines (i.e., *E. coli* J-5) in dairy cattle has been shown to reduce the incidence and severity of clinical coliform mastitis [29].
B. *S. aureus* is the most common cause of contagious mastitis in dairy cattle [30]. *S. aureus* usually causes subclinical mastitis and chronic mastitis with high somatic cell counts [31]. *S. aureus* has several mechanisms enabling it to evade the host immune response, and intramammary infection with *S. aureus* typically results in a very moderate host response [24, 27]. This leads to a limited cytokine response to *S. aureus,* which aids in establishing chronicity. In addition, *S. aureus* produces leukotoxin and can survive in and destroy phagocytic cells [32–34]. This leads to evasion of the immune system, chronicity of infection, and difficulty in removing the bacteria from infected quarters.

Conclusion

Early detection and recognition of the varied causes of mastitis are key to the control of the disorder. Immune responses stimulated by damage to the mammary gland are complex and may depend on the stage of lactation and the microbe involved in the initiation of the inflammation. The balance required to limit infections and minimize inflammation drives a unique blend of cells, cytokines, and chemokines. As more is learned about the pathogenesis of unique forms of mastitis, targeted therapeutic interventions, and the role of specific immune mediators, the prevention and treatment of mastitis will likely improve.

Your Case

The manager of a 1200-cow pasture-based dairy in the Southeast United States calls after hours to report that three cows in peak lactation were found recumbent by the night milking crew. The cows are unable to rise, and the manager requests that you examine and treat the cows. It is August, and the weather has been extremely hot with severe thunderstorms for the last 24 h.

Upon arrival, you find three cows, second and third lactation, unable to rise in the pasture. Despite good pasture management, the rain has caused some muddy areas in the pasture. The cows are dehydrated with temperatures ranging from 104.6 to 106 °F. The cows are 45–60 days in milk. With some assistance, you roll the cows to their sides and find that each has an extremely swollen quarter. The milk is a brownish-colored fluid and is hot.

Questions

1. What is your tentative diagnosis? How do you confirm it?
2. How do you treat the recumbent cows? What do you anticipate for an outcome?
3. Why is the dairy experiencing this problem?
4. The following day, the dairy finds two more cows with hard quarters, elevated temperatures, and anorexia. What is your course of action to prevent new cases?

Additional Readings

1. Quintas H, Margatho G, Rodríguez-Estévez V, Simões J. Understanding mastitis in goats (I): etiopathophysiological particularities. In: Simões J, Gutiérrez C, editors. Sustainable goat production in adverse environments: volume I. Cham: Springer; 2017. https://doi.org/10.1007/978-3-319-71855-2_18.
2. Gelasakis AI, Mavrogianni VS, Petridis IG, Vasileiou NGC, Fthenakis GC. Mastitis in sheep—the last 10 years and the future of research. Vet Microbiol. 2015;181(1–2):136–46. ISSN 0378-1135. https://doi.org/10.1016/j.vetmic.2015.07.009.
3. Sordillo LM. Mammary gland immunobiology and resistance to mastitis. Vet Clin North Am Food Anim Pract. 2018;34(3):507–23. https://doi.org/10.1016/j.cvfa.2018.07.005. PMID: 30316507.
4. Sordillo LM, Streicher KL. Mammary gland immunity and mastitis susceptibility. J Mammary Gland Biol Neoplasia. 2002;7(2):135–46. https://doi.org/10.1023/a:1020347818725. PMID: 12463736.
5. Stanek P, Żółkiewski P, Januś E. A review on mastitis in dairy cows research: current status and future perspectives. Agriculture. 2024;14(8):1292. https://doi.org/10.3390/agriculture14081292.
6. Kiyono H, Kweon MN, Hiroi T, Takahashi I. The mucosal immune system: from specialized immune defense to inflammation and allergy. Acta Odontol Scand. 2001;59(3):145–53. https://doi.org/10.1080/000163501750266738. PMID: 11501883.
7. Chase C, Kaushik RS. System mucosal immune of cattle: all immune responses begin here. Vet Clin North Am Food Anim Pract. 2019;35(3):431–45.

8. Aitken SL, Corl CM, Sordillo LM. Immunopathology of mastitis: insights into disease recognition and resolution. J Mammary Gland Biol Neoplasia. 2011;16(4):291–304. https://doi.org/10.1007/s10911-011-9230-4. Epub 2011 Sep 22. PMID: 21938490.
9. Ezzat Alnakip M, Quintela-Baluja M, Böhme K. The immunology of mammary gland of dairy ruminants between healthy and inflammatory conditions. J Vet Med. 2014;31. https://doi.org/10.1155/2014/659801.
10. Rinaldi M, Li RW, Bannerman DD, Daniels KM, Evock-Clover C, Silva MVB, Paape MJ, Van Ryssen B, Burvenich C, Capuco AV. A sentinel function for teat tissues in dairy cows: dominant innate immune response elements define early response to E. coli mastitis. Funct Integr Genomics. 2010;10:21–38. https://doi.org/10.1007/s10142-009-0133-z.
11. Bronzo V, Lopreiato V, Riva F, Amadori M, Curone G, Addis MF, Cremonesi P, Moroni P, Trevisi E, Castiglioni B. The role of innate immune response and microbiome in resilience of dairy cattle to disease: the mastitis model. Animals (Basel). 2020;10(8):1397. https://doi.org/10.3390/ani10081397. PMID: 32796642; PMCID: PMC7459693.
12. Paape MJ, Shafer-Weaver K, Capuco AV, Van Oostveldt K, Burvenich C. Immune surveillance of mammary tissue by phagocytic cells. Adv Exp Med Biol. 2000;480:259–77. https://doi.org/10.1007/0-306-46832-8_31. [DOI] [PubMed] [Google Scholar].
13. Denis M, Parlane NA, Lacy-Hulbert SJ, Summers EL, Buddle BM, Wedlock DN. Bactericidal activity of macrophages against streptococcus uberis is different in mammary gland secretions of lactating and drying off cows. Vet Immunol Immunopathol. 2006;114:111–20. https://doi.org/10.1016/j.vetimm.2006.08.001.
14. Paape MJ, Bannermann DD, Zhao X. The bovine neutrophil: structure and function in blood and milk. Vet Res. 2003;34:597–627. https://doi.org/10.1051/vetres:2003024.
15. Diwakar R, Kumar P, Deora A, Sharma H, Sharma S, Mittal D, Bhanot V, Prakash A, Yadav R. Bovine mastitis: a review. Middle-East J Sci Res. 2020;28(6):497–507.
16. Taylor BC, Dellinger JD, Cullor JS, Stott JL. Bovine milk lymphocytes display the phenotype of memory T cells and are predominantly CD8+. Cell Ther Immunol. 1994;156:245–53. https://doi.org/10.1006/cimm.1994.1169. [DOI] [PubMed] [Google Scholar].
17. Sordillo LM. Factors affecting mammary gland immunity and mastitis susceptibility. Livest Prod Sci. 2005;9(1–2):89–99. ISSN 0301-6226. https://doi.org/10.1016/j.livprodsci.2005.10.017.
18. Tucker T, Cunha P, Gilbert FB, Rambault M, Reis Santos K, Remot A, Germon P, Rainard P, Martins RP. Bovine blood and milk T-cell subsets in distinct states of activation and differentiation during subclinical Staphylococcus aureus mastitis. J Reprod Immunol. 2023;156:103826. ISSN 0165-0378. https://doi.org/10.1016/j.jri.2023.103826.
19. Lohova E, Pilmane M, Šerstņova K, Melderis I, Gontar Ł, Kochański M, Prieto-Simón B. Analysis of inflammatory and regulatory cytokines in the milk of dairy cows with mastitis: a comparative study with healthy animals. Immunol Investig. 2024;53(8):1397–421. https://doi.org/10.1080/08820139.2024.2404623.
20. Riollet C, Rainard P, Poutrel B. Kinetics of cells and cytokines during immune-mediated inflammation in the mammary gland of cows systemically immunized with Staphylococcus aureus α-toxin. J Inflamm Res. 2000;49:486–96.
21. Vitenberga-Verza Z, Pilmane M, Šerstņova K, Melderis I, Gontar Ł, Kochański M, Drutowska A, Maróti G, Prieto-Simón B. Identification of inflammatory and regulatory cytokines IL-1α-, IL-4-, IL-6-, IL-12-, IL-13-, IL-17A-, tnf-α-, and ifn-γ-producing cells in the milk of dairy cows with subclinical and clinical mastitis. Pathogens. 2022;11(3):372. https://doi.org/10.3390/pathogens11030372.
22. Paul WE. Interleukin-4: a prototypic immunoregulatory lymphokine. Blood. 1991;77(9):1859. https://doi.org/10.1182/blood.V77.9.1859.1859.
23. Goulart DB, Mellata M. Escherichia coli mastitis in dairy cattle: etiology, diagnosis, and treatment challenges. Front Microbiol. 2022;13:928346. https://doi.org/10.3389/fmicb.2022.928346. PMID: 35875575; PMCID: PMC9301288.

24. Tong X, Barkema HW, Nobrega DB, Xu C, Han B, Zhang C, Yang J, Li X, Gao J. Virulence of bacteria causing mastitis in dairy cows: a literature review. Microorganisms. 2025;13(1):167. https://doi.org/10.3390/microorganisms13010167. PMID: 39858935; PMCID: PMC11767654.
25. Hagiwara S, Mori K, Okada H, Oikawa S, Nagahata H. Acute Escherichia coli mastitis in dairy cattle: diagnostic parameters associated with poor prognosis. J Vet Med Sci. 2014;76(11):1431–6. https://doi.org/10.1292/jvms.13-0610. Epub 2014 Jul 24. PMID: 25056677; PMCID: PMC4272974.
26. Burvenich C, Bannerman DD, Lippolis JD, Peelman L, Nonnecke BJ, Kehrli ME, Paape MJ. Cumulative physiological events influence the inflammatory response of the bovine udder to Escherichia coli infections during the transition period. J Dairy Sci. 2007;90(Supplement):E39–54. ISSN 0022-0302. https://doi.org/10.3168/jds.2006-696.
27. Schukken YH, Günther J, Fitzpatrick J, Fontaine MC, Goetze L, Holst O, Leigh J, Petzl W, Schuberth HJ, Sipka A, Smith DG, Quesnell R, Watts J, Yancey R, Zerbe H, Gurjar A, Zadoks RN, Seyfert HM, members of the Pfizer mastitis research consortium. Host-response patterns of intramammary infections in dairy cows. Vet Immunol Immunopathol. 2011;144(3–4):270–89. https://doi.org/10.1016/j.vetimm.2011.08.022. Epub 2011 Sep 10. PMID: 21955443.
28. van Amersfoort ES, Van Berkel TJ, Kuiper J. Receptors, mediators, and mechanisms involved in bacterial sepsis and septic shock. Clin Microbiol Rev. 2003;16:379–414.
29. Johnzon CF, Dahlberg J, Gustafson AM, Waernlda W, Moazzami AA, Östensson K, Gunnar P. The effect of lipopolysaccharide-induced experimental bovine mastitis on clinical parameters, inflammatory markers, and the metabolome: a kinetic approach. Front Immunol. 2018;9:1487. Published 2018 Jun 25. https://doi.org/10.3389/fimmu.2018.01487.
30. Gonzalez RN, Cullor JS, Jasper DE, Farver TB, Bushnell RB, Oliver MN. Prevention of clinical coliform mastitis in dairy cows by a mutant Escherichia coli vaccine. Can J Vet Res. 1989;53:301–5.
31. Kerro Dego O, Vidlund J. Staphylococcal mastitis in dairy cows. Front Vet Sci. 2024;11:1356259. https://doi.org/10.3389/fvets.2024.1356259. PMID: 38863450; PMCID: PMC11165426.
32. Bannerman DD, Paape MJ, Lee JW, Zhao X, Hope JC, Rainard P. Escherichia coli and Staphylococcus aureus elicit differential innate immune responses following intramammary infection. Clin Diagn Lab Immunol. 2004;11(3):463–72. https://doi.org/10.1128/CDLI.11.3.463-472.2004.
33. Vann JM, Proctor RA. Cytotoxic effects of ingested Staphylococcus aureus on bovine endothelial cells: role of S. aureus α-hemolysin. Microb Pathog. 1988;4:443–53. https://doi.org/10.1016/0882-4010(88)90029-0.
34. Cai J, Li J, Zhou Y, Wang J, Li J, Cui L, Meng X, Zhu G, Wang H. Staphylococcus aureus facilitates its survival in bovine macrophages by blocking autophagic flux. J Cell Mol Med. 2020;24(6):3460–8. https://doi.org/10.1111/jcmm.15027. Epub 2020 Jan 29. PMID: 31997584; PMCID: PMC7131951.

Immunology of the Respiratory Tract 12

Abstract

Anatomical and physiological species-specific differences make cattle more prone to developing respiratory disease than other species. They have a smaller lung capacity, which requires a higher rate of breathing compared to other species. Their lung anatomy is prone to allowing pathogens deeper into in lungs, which have poor collateral ventilation, predisposing cattle to emphysema. The mucociliary escalator provides barrier function in the respiratory tract; it can be disrupted by environmental and microbial factors. The innate immune response in the respiratory tract comprises phagocytic cells, pro-inflammatory cytokines, anti-microbial peptides, and other soluble factors. The adaptive immune response in the respiratory tract is performed by mucosa-associated lymphoid tissue and other secondary lymphoid organs, including tonsils and lymph nodes. Disease-sparing in the respiratory tract is accomplished by local and systemic antibody and cell-mediated immunity (CMI) responses.

Keywords

Bovine respiratory disease complex (BRDC) · Mucociliary escalator · Mucous-associated lymphoid tissue (MALT) · IgG1 · Dysbiosis

Key Concepts

- *Species-specific differences* in anatomy and physiology make cattle more prone to developing respiratory disease than other species.
- The *mucociliary escalator* provides barrier function in the respiratory tract; it can be disrupted by environmental and microbial factors.
- The *innate immune response* in the respiratory tract comprises phagocytic cells, pro-inflammatory cytokines, anti-microbial peptides, and other soluble factors.

J. Ellis, V. Cortese, *Practical Bovine Immunology*,
https://doi.org/10.1007/978-3-032-15031-8_12

- The *adaptive immune response* in the respiratory tract is performed by mucosa-associated lymphoid tissue and other secondary lymphoid organs, including tonsils and lymph nodes.
- *Disease-sparing* in the respiratory tract is accomplished by local and systemic antibody and cell-mediated immunity responses.

Why Are Cattle More Prone to Developing Respiratory Disease Than Other Species?

The bovine respiratory disease complex (BRDC) is the most persistent, economically important disease in cattle, certainly in feedlot cattle. There are a plethora of management factors that contribute to the high prevalence of BRDC. They are beyond the scope of this text, but it is important to remember the anatomical and physiological factors that make cattle particularly prone to developing pneumonia compared to other veterinary species [1]. Bovine lungs are disproportionately undersized relative to their body size. For example, horses may have a lung capacity of over 50 L, whereas in an adult cow, it is only about 13 L, on average. This means that they have a relatively small tidal volume of about 3–6 L, and to meet their high oxygen demand, they compensate for this by a relatively higher resting respiratory rate of around 20, compared to 15 in a dog and 8 in a horse. Quite simply, more breaths per minute provide more chance for inhaling noxious particles such as microbes or dust. Moreover, ruminants, including cattle, have a unique bronchial anatomy in which the right cranial lobe branches directly from the trachea. This provides a more direct pathway to the lung for microbes, such as *Mannheimia hemolytica*, leading to the common occurrence of bronchopneumonia. Micro-anatomically, cattle have a comparatively low alveolar surface area and reduced capillary density, which limits gas exchange. They also have relatively thick interlobular septa that compartmentalize the lungs, making them prone to develop the lobar pneumonia that is typical of *M. hemolytica* infection. Importantly, as well, they have poor collateral ventilation because of reduced inter-alveolar and inter-airway connections. Because of this deficiency, they have difficulty compensating for local damage to the small airways and alveoli. This makes them particularly prone to develop atelectasis (collapse) and interstitial emphysema (air leakage and trapping) as a result of bovine respiratory syncytial virus (BRSV) infection or pneumointoxication due to rumen metabolites such as 3-methylindole, both of which damage bronchiolar and pulmonary parenchymal (type 1) epithelial cells, resulting in broncho-interstitial pneumonia [2]. Necrotic bronchiolar and alveolar cells, together with inflammatory debris, can act as a one-way valve of sorts, letting air in, but not effectively out. This can result in tachypnea and expiratory dyspnea (puffing) that is typical of acute respiratory distress syndrome, such as in BRSV infections.

What Are the Components of the Innate Immune System in the Respiratory Tract in Cattle?

As in other organ systems in cattle and other mammals, the innate immune system of the respiratory tract comprises physical and physiological barriers, cellular defenses, and soluble factors that act as a first line of defense against invaders [3, 4]. The long nasal cavity of cattle is lined by tortuous turbinates that filter, warm, and humidify the air. Tight epithelial junctions maintain a sealed barrier between cells. The so-called "mucociliary escalator" begins in the nasal cavity and extends through to the bronchioles. It comprises ciliated epithelial cells, goblet cells, and submucosal glands that produce mucous. Inhaled particles are trapped in the mucous and then removed by the rhythmic upward movement of the cilia. Reflexive coughing and sneezing mechanically expel microbes and irritants such as dust.

Numerous cells can contribute to an innate immune response in the respiratory tract. Neutrophils and alveolar macrophages can phagocytize and enzymatically destroy microbes. Neutrophils also release granules containing perforin and granzyme that have cytotoxic activities on microbes. Natural killer cells and γδ T cells are both of lymphocyte lineage and can recognize infected cells in a variety of ways, but unlike other lymphocytes, in a non-Major Histocompatibility Complex-restricted fashion. They, like neutrophils, release perforin and granzyme-containing granules to kill infected cells and secrete a variety of cytokines. Dendritic cells are scattered among the airway epithelium and in the submucosa and alveolar spaces. They sample those microenvironments for microbial invaders primarily by recognizing pathogen-associated molecular patterns (PAMP) and can secrete a variety of cytokines in response. Infection can upregulate the expression of various receptors for these ligands, the PRR, on and in a variety of cells, including dendritic cells.

Many soluble mediators are part of the first line of defense in the respiratory tract. Proinflammatory cytokines, interleukin (IL)-1, IL-6, tumor necrosis factor (TNF-α), are produced by many cell types, including macrophages, dendritic cells, neutrophils, and, sometimes, epithelial cells. These promote inflammation and recruit and activate other immune cells. Chemokines, notably CXCL8 or IL-8, are produced by macrophages, dendritic cells, and epithelial cells and attract neutrophils and other leukocytes to the sites of microbial invasion. Type I interferons (IFN-α and IFN-β) are produced by infected epithelial cells and dendritic cells. They have direct antiviral effects and activate immune cells and enhance antigen presentation. Antimicrobial peptides, notably defensins and cathelicidins, are produced by epithelial cells and neutrophils. They can directly kill bacteria, fungi, and some viruses. Lactoferrin and lysozyme are other products of neutrophils and epithelial cells. Lactoferrin disrupts membranes and sequesters iron, affecting a broad range of bacteria, fungi, and viruses. The enzyme, lysozyme, cleaves the peptidoglycan of Gram-positive bacteria. Complement proteins, in addition to being produced primarily by the liver, can be produced locally by many cell types in the respiratory tract. C3 and C5 and their cleavage products are probably the most important factors in that cascade in the respiratory tract, where they act as opsonins, chemoattractants, and promoters of inflammation. Surfactant is a complex mixture of lipids and proteins that is secreted primarily by type II epithelial cells in the lung. In addition to its critical role in maintaining normal respiratory physiology, two of its proteins, SP-A and SP-D, can bind invaders and enhance clearance by alveolar macrophages.

In addition to playing a protective role, especially in the early stages, the innate response plays a key pathogenic role in BRD [4, 5]. Overproduction of pro-inflammatory cytokines in response to increased presence of various viral and bacterial Pathogen-associated molecular patterns exacerbates inflammation beyond protective levels. Much of the sickness behavior in calves with bacterial pneumonias can be explained on the basis of the systemic effects of this pulmonary "cytokine storm." Increased amounts of cytokines and chemokines also recruit excess neutrophils to sites of infection [4, 5]. Neutrophils and their many enzymes contribute to the tissue damage that is characteristic of BRD. This was classically demonstrated in *M. hemolytica* infections in neutrophil-depleted calves; they had less severe lesions than normal calves [6]. More recently, it has been suggested that the variation in clinical response and lung disease in BRD-effected cattle could be attributable to individual differences in the (innate) inflammatory response to the same infection [5]. Cattle with less pronounced inflammatory responses to respiratory infection have less disease. In other words, the inflammatory response to infection is the disease. Overall, acknowledging the pathologic role of the innate inflammatory response in BRD justifies the concept of using anti-inflammatory drugs, like non-steroidal anti-inflammatory drugs, as adjunct therapy together with antibiotics; however, so far, there are few data to support this approach [7, 8]. This could be a matter of dosage, frequency, or the timing of treatment, and warrants further investigation.

How Do Invaders and Environmental Factors Compromise the Innate Immune System in the Respiratory Tract in Cattle?

Microbial infections and environmental factors can act synergistically to impair innate immune function and predispose to BRD [3, 4]. A combination and persistence of stressors, such as weaning, transportation, and overcrowding, can increase cortisol levels and suppress innate (and adaptive) immune function. Poor air quality resulting from high levels of ammonia, dust, or extremes in humidity or dryness can damage the respiratory epithelium and impair mucociliary function. Similarly, sudden changes or extremes in temperature can reduce immune function and increase susceptibility to infection. In addition to these environmental factors, nutritional deficiencies, notably of vitamin A, E, or trace minerals (such as zinc and selenium), can affect epithelial integrity and function and suppress immune function. Abrupt changes in diet can influence the production of pneumotoxic ruminal metabolites.

What Is the Role of Passive Immunity (Colostrum) in the Respiratory Tract in Calves?

In contrast to some other species, notably humans, the predominant immunoglobulin in colostrum is IgG1. It is absorbed and re-secreted onto mucosal surfaces, including the respiratory tract [9]. In contrast, IgG2 is at a lower concentration in colostrum and is not effectively re-secreted. Being particularly effective at neutralizing viruses and bacterial toxins, IgG1 can contribute significantly to reducing adherence and colonization of pathogens, resulting in sparing of disease, for example, in BRSV infections [10]. From a management perspective, the respiratory disease-sparing effects of passively transferred immunoglobulins to the calf can be enhanced by perinatal vaccination of the dam [10]. However, these antibodies are only protective against pneumonia in the young calf.

What Are the Components of the Adaptive Immune System in the Respiratory Tract in Cattle and How Do They Combat Microbial Invaders?

Immune defense of the respiratory tract involves both mucosal and systemic adaptive immune responses [4]. Beginning in the nasal cavity and extending into the lung, there is an extensive network of submucosal lymphoid tissue collectively known as mucous-associated lymphoid tissue (MALT). This is further subdivided into nasal-associated lymphoid tissue and bronchus-associated lymphoid tissue. This tissue contains a full range of the players in adaptive immunity, including "helper" (CD4+) and "killer" (CD8+) T cells, B cells, and plasma cells [11, 12]. These cells are found dispersed in the submucosa and in organized lymphoid follicles, often with germinal centers, where B cell maturation and class-switching (of antibodies) occur. As well, there are many antigen-presenting cells; mostly dendritic cells that express high amounts of Major Histocompatibility Complex-2 molecules, indicative of their efficiency in stimulating lymphocytes. The isotypes of the antibodies in B cells and plasma cells vary somewhat with location (in the respiratory tract) and health status. In the nose and upper airways, IgA predominates, whereas in the lower respiratory tract (LTR), IgG1 and IgG2 predominate. Although MALT is considered secondary lymphoid tissue, cattle also have numerous discrete secondary lymphoid organs that are closely associated with the respiratory tract. They surveil and respond to the respiratory microenvironment. In the upper respiratory tract (UTR), cattle have five different types of tonsils [13]. Some of them, notably the large pharyngeal tonsil, located at the caudal end of the pharyngeal septum, are lined by respiratory (pseudo-stratified columnar) epithelium in which viruses, such as BRSV, can replicate. Proteomic analysis (characterization of proteins present) indicates that these tonsils can react to respiratory infections with a wide range of both antibody and cell-mediated immunity responses [14]. In both upper and lower portions of the respiratory tract, lymph drains in afferent lymphatics to numerous directly associated lymph nodes, of which there are five main sets. Similar to the tonsils, transcriptomic analysis (characterization of mRNA transcripts present) of lymph nodes from cattle with respiratory disease, such as the bronchial nodes, reveals that hundreds of genes associated with antibody and cell-mediated immunity can be upregulated in response to viral and bacterial infections [15, 16]. Resulting antibodies and T cells can then recirculate back to the lungs. At the feedlot or dairy, graphic morphologic evidence of these responses, in virtually any case of clinical respiratory disease, can be routinely observed at postmortem by simply slicing through tonsils and respiratory tract-associated lymph nodes. There will usually be marked hyperplasia with large prominent lymphoid follicles (B cell areas in the cortex) and an interspersed expanded paracortex (T cell area). From a practical standpoint, envisioning the myriads of respiratory lymphoid elements, it is easy to understand why intranasal administration of vaccines can stimulate a broad range of adaptive immune responses that can help protect all levels of the respiratory tract from disease.

Beyond the respiratory tract itself, systemic immune responses can also play a role in protecting the respiratory tract [4]. Although immunoglobulins are large molecules that are generally confined to the plasma, there are both passive and active mechanisms that allow the transfer of IgG from circulation across the alveolar barrier. These antibodies may have been produced in local or distant lymph nodes, or in other secondary lymphoid organs, such as the spleen, and entered the circulating blood. Under normal conditions in healthy lungs, the capillary-alveolar junction is tight. Nevertheless, small amounts of IgG can passively diffuse into alveolar spaces by transudation. There is also active transport of IgG into the lung. This is accomplished through the expression of the neonatal Fc receptor on pulmonary capillary endothelial cells and alveolar epithelial cells [17]. These receptors bind the Fc portion of IgG (the base of the "Y"). Then, the bound antibody is internalized via endocytosis and transported across the cell to the other side, ending up in the alveolar space. Finally, there is inflammation-enhanced permeability, which accounts for the most extra-vascular antibody. Proinflammatory cytokines such as TNF-α, IL-1, and IL-6 cause the tight junctions between endothelial cells and epithelial cells to loosen and become leaky. This results in the exudation of large amounts of immunoglobulins as well as neutrophils and lymphocytes from the bloodstream into the pulmonary interstitial and alveolar spaces. There is also inflammation-enhanced recruitment of B cells and plasma cells that further increase the amount of locally produced IgG in respiratory secretions. The best practical circumstantial evidence for the involvement of systemic immune responses in protecting the respiratory tract is the ability of parenterally administered inactivated [18] and subunit [19] vaccines, which do not contain microbes that can replicate locally in the lung, to confer disease-sparing immunity to infection.

Regardless of the source, mucosal or systemic, antibody responses in the respiratory tract have sometimes been measured as a correlate of immune protection, often in the context of studies of vaccine efficacy. Correlations between both IgA and IgG with clinical protection have been documented [4]. Functional studies of pulmonary antigen-specific T cell responses, particularly "killer" T (CD8+) responses, have been less frequently measured. Largely, the reason for the relative lack of data on pathogen-specific immune responses in the respiratory tract is simply a sampling issue; it is a lot easier to collect blood (serum) than it is to conduct a broncho-pulmonary lavage to obtain lung-resident cells and secretions. It can also be problematic to collect consistent samples of nasal secretions. Measurement of antigen-specific respiratory CD8+ cytotoxic T cells is further complicated by the necessity of having Major Histocompatibility Complex-matched "target cells," remembering that these T cells can only recognize a microbe if parts of it (peptides) are presented by their own Major Histocompatibility Complex-1 molecules on the surface of an infected cell. This essentially means deriving cell cultures from each calf to be tested [20]. Nevertheless, it is highly likely, based on the scant evidence there is, that pulmonary cell-mediated immunity responses, including both cytolytic CD8+ T cell responses, as well as cytokine production by CD4+ T cells, are important in the recovery from viral [20] and intracellular bacterial infections [21].

What Is the Role of the Microbiome in Affecting Respiratory Immune Responses in Cattle?

It is now generally acknowledged that the microbiome of the respiratory tract, comprising the microbes, their genes, and how they interact in the (respiratory) environment, contributes to, or determines, respiratory "health," which is observed as clinical "normalcy" [22, 23]. There are considered to be two distinct and different microbiomes in the respiratory tract: one above and including the larynx, the UTR microbiome, and one below the larynx, the LTR microbiome.

A critical characteristic of (respiratory) health is thought to be homeostasis of the microbiome, a stable and balanced state. Two measures relating to this homeostasis are richness and diversity. Richness refers to the number of different microbes in a given sample or environment, whereas diversity indicates how evenly individual microbes are distributed in that community. A common measure of microbial diversity that accounts for both richness and how evenly individual microbes are represented is the Shannon index. This is calculated by a computer-driven analysis of massive amounts of metagenomic, that is, sequencing, data, without the need for culturing. Based on this, the UTR microbiome is more *diverse than the lower respiratory microbiome and, in fact, usually contains bacteria, such as M. hemolyica, Pasteurella multocida, Histophilus somni,* and *Mycoplasma bovis.* These same microbes are commonly implicated as pneumonic pathogens, most convincingly by immunohistochemical staining of BRD-effected lung tissue that reveals the pronounced presence of one or more of them in typical lesions [24]. Importantly, in a "normal" bovid, with a homeostatic microbiome, these are commonly resident commensals in the UTR, serving normal physiologic functions, or at least apparently doing no harm. When the homeostasis of the respiratory microbiome becomes disrupted or imbalanced, a state of dysbiosis occurs, often leading to a state of decreased diversity and associated BRD. Co-factors fostering this change include stress and environmental factors, antibiotic use, and changes in diet and nutrition, essentially, many components of modern livestock production. Acknowledging that there are conflicting data related to sampling, timing of sampling, and inclusion criteria, it remains unclear if decreased diversity predisposes cattle to BRD, or, vice versa, the decreased diversity in cattle with BRD is due to disease development—a largely unresolved question of cause and effect [19].

Conceptually, it is easy to imagine that the microbiome interacts with the immune system and modulates responses [18, 19]. The large numbers and amount of Pathogen-associated molecular patterns present in a complex microbial community indicate how much signaling could occur between the microbiome and the respiratory immune system. But, unfortunately, there is limited data from cattle studies to indicate, mechanistically, how the microbiome(s) specifically influences the immune response in the bovine respiratory tract. Therefore, practical, evidence-based applications deriving from the burgeoning data concerning the microbiome(s) of the respiratory tract remain largely to be determined.

Your Case

History

In early spring, a respiratory disease outbreak emerged on a commercial dairy farm in the Midwest. The farm housed around 250 milking cows and maintained a group of 60 replacement heifers. Calves were separated from their dams within 2 h of birth and fed 2 L of colostrum, either by bottle or esophageal feeder. However, the farm did not routinely assess colostrum quality, and no serum total protein testing was done to confirm passive transfer. Calves were housed individually in outdoor hutches with straw bedding and were fed milk replacer twice daily, with free access to water and calf starter. The outbreak began subtly, with a few calves showing mild respiratory signs, but within 10 days, the majority of the group was affected.

Clinical Findings

The affected calves, all around 3 months old, began showing signs of respiratory distress. Most had fevers ranging from 103.5 to 105.8 °F and were breathing rapidly, with rates between 60 and 80 breaths per minute. Harsh lung sounds were audible on auscultation, and many calves had a serous to mucopurulent nasal discharge. Coughing was common, and several calves showed reduced appetites and poor weight gain. Four calves were severely affected, displaying open-mouth breathing, cyanotic mucous membranes, and eventually becoming recumbent. Despite supportive care, these calves died within 48 hours of showing severe symptoms.

Necropsy Findings

Necropsies were performed on two of the deceased calves. The most striking findings were in the lungs, where 40–60% of the cranioventral lung lobes were consolidated. There was also evidence of fibrinous pleuritis, and the tracheal mucosa appeared reddened and inflamed. The mediastinal lymph nodes were enlarged. Histopathological examination revealed a suppurative bronchopneumonia, with heavy infiltration of neutrophils in the alveoli and bronchioles, and fibrin exudate lining the pleural surfaces.

Diagnostic Data

To investigate the underlying cause, serum samples were retrospectively collected from the affected group. The average serum total protein was 4.8 g/dL, with 70% of calves falling below the 5.2 g/dL threshold—confirming a widespread failure of passive transfer. Nasal swabs and lung tissue samples were submitted for PCR testing. The results identified *Pasteurella multocida*, *Mannheimia haemolytica*, and BRSV as the primary pathogens involved. Tests for IBR, PI3, and *Mycoplasma bovis* were negative. Antibiotic sensitivity testing showed that the bacterial isolates were susceptible to florfenicol and ceftiofur.

Veterinary Interventions

Upon confirmation of the outbreak, the veterinary team implemented several immediate and long-term interventions. Affected calves were isolated, and metaphylactic treatment with florfenicol was administered to the entire group. Severely ill calves received ceftiofur and flunixin meglumine to reduce inflammation and fever. Supportive care included oral electrolytes and anti-inflammatory medications. The farm also made significant changes to its management practices. Colostrum quality began to be assessed using a Brix refractometer, and the volume fed was increased to 4 L within the first 6 h of life. Serum total protein testing was introduced as a routine check at 48 h post-birth. Additionally, the vaccination protocol was updated to include intranasal BRSV and *M. haemolytica* vaccines administered at 1 week of age.

Outcome

The outbreak resulted in the death of four calves, representing a 20% mortality rate within the affected group. Fourteen of the 20 calves showed clinical signs, but the majority responded well to treatment. No new cases were reported after 3 weeks, indicating that the interventions were effective in controlling the outbreak. The farm's revised colostrum and vaccination protocols have since helped reduce the incidence of respiratory disease in subsequent calf cohorts.

Questions for You

1. What does a BRIX value indicate, and how is it measured?
2. How is total serum protein in calves determined? How does it relate to IgG concentrations? What is considered evidence of adequate passive transfer?
3. Why are calves with bacterial pneumonia "sick," and what is the role of the innate immune system in "sickness behavior"?
4. Why are intranasal vaccines potentially more efficacious than injectable vaccines, especially in young calves?

Additional Readings

1. Veit HP, Farrell RL. The anatomy and physiology of the bovine respiratory system relating to pulmonary disease. Cornell Vet. 1978;68(4):555–81. PMID: 361341.
2. Bingham HR, Morley PS, Wittum TE, Bray TM, West KH, Slemons RD, Ellis JA, Haines DM, Levy MA, Sarver CF, Saville WJ, Cortese VS. Synergistic effects of concurrent challenge with bovine respiratory syncytial virus and 3-methylindole in calves. Am J Vet Res. 1999;60(5):563–70. PMID: 10328425.
3. Ackermann MR, Derscheid R, Roth JA. Innate immunology of bovine respiratory disease. Vet Clin North Am Food Anim Pract. 2010;26(2):215–28. https://doi.org/10.1016/j.cvfa.2010.03.001. Epub 2010 May 14. PMID: 20619180; PMCID: PMC2904317.
4. McGill JL, Sacco RE. The immunology of bovine respiratory disease: recent advancements. Vet Clin N Am Food Anim Pract. 2020;36:333–48. https://doi.org/10.1016/j.cvfa.2020.03.002.
5. Bassel LL, Tabatabaei S, Caswell JL. Host tolerance to infection with the bacteria that cause bovine respiratory disease. Vet Clin N Am Food Anim Pract. 2020;36:349–59. https://doi.org/10.1016/j.cvfa.2020.03.003.
6. Slocombe RF, Malark J, Ingersoll R, Derksen FJ, Robinson NE. Importance of neutrophils in the pathogenesis of acute pneumonic pasteurellosis in calves. Am J Vet Res. 1985 Nov;46(11):2253–8. PMID: 4073635.
7. Ferree LA, Edwards-Callaway LN, Roman-Muniz IN, Coetzee JHF, Applegate TJ, Ollivett TL, Cramer MC. Oral meloxicam given as an ancillary treatment at respiratory disease diagnosis was not associated with growth, clinical scores, or ultrasound scores in preweaned dairy calves. J Am Vet Med Assoc. 2023;261(11):1716–23.
8. Hägglund S, Laloy E, Alvarez I, Guo Y, Hallbrink Ågren G, Yazdan Panah H, Widgren A, Bergquist J, Hillström A, Baillif V, Saias L, Dubourdeau M, Timsit E, Valarcher JF. Effects of early treatment with nonsteroidal anti-inflammatory drugs (NSAIDs) on the bronchoalveolar lavage proteome and oxylipids during bovine respiratory syncytial virus (BRSV) infection. PLoS One. 2024;19(11):e0309609. https://doi.org/10.1371/journal.pone.0309609. PMID: 39546485; PMCID: PMC11567528.
9. Ellis JA, Chamorro MF, Lacoste S, Gow SP, Haines DM. Bovine respiratory syncytial virus-specific IgG-1 in nasal secretions of colostrum-fed neonatal calves. Can Vet J. 2018;59(5):505–8. PMID: 29904203; PMCID: PMC5901845.
10. Meyer G, Foret-Lucas C, Delverdier M, Cuquemelle A, Secula A, Cassard H. Protection against bovine respiratory syncytial virus afforded by maternal antibodies from cows immunized with an inactivated vaccine. Vaccines (Basel). 2023;11(1):141. https://doi.org/10.3390/vaccines11010141. PMID: 36679988; PMCID: PMC9864491.
11. Thomasmeyer A, Reineking W, Hewicker-Trautwein M. Histological and immunohistochemical characterization of mucous-associated lymphoid tissue and antigen presenting cells in trachea and lung of cattle. Anat Histol Embryol. 2023;52:989–1002. https://doi.org/10.1111/ahe.12959.
12. Meek HC, Stenfeldt C, Arzt J. Morphological and phenotypic characteristics of the bovine nasopharyngeal mucosa and associated lymphoid tissue. J Comp Pathol. 2022;198:62–79.
13. Casteleyn C, Breugelmans S, Simoens P, Van den Broeck W. The tonsils revisited: review of the anatomical localization and histological characteristics of the tonsils of domestic and laboratory animals. Clin Dev Immunol. 2011;2011:472460. https://doi.org/10.1155/2011/472460. Epub 2011 Aug 21. PMID: 21869895; PMCID: PMC3159307.
14. Gray D, Ellis JA, Gow SP, Lacoste SR, Allan GM, Mooney MH. Profiling of local disease-sparing responses to bovine respiratory syncytial virus in intranasally vaccinated and challenged calves. J Proteome. 2019;204:103397, ISSN 1874-3919. https://doi.org/10.1016/j.jprot.2019.103397.
15. Tizioto PC, Kim J, Seabury CM, Schnabel RD, Gershwin LJ, Van Eenennaam AL, Toaff-Rosenstein R, Neibergs HL; Bovine Respiratory Disease Complex Coordinated Agricultural Project Research Team; Taylor JF. Immunological response to single pathogen challenge with

agents of the bovine respiratory disease complex: an RNA-sequence analysis of the bronchial lymph node transcriptome. PLoS One. 2015;10(6):e0131459. https://doi.org/10.1371/journal.pone.0131459. PMID: 26121276; PMCID: PMC4484807.

16. Johnston D, Earley B, McCabe MS, Kim J, Taylor JF, Lemon K, McMenamy M, Duffy C, Cosby SL, Waters SM. Elucidation of the host bronchial lymph node miRNA transcriptome response to bovine respiratory syncytial virus. Front Genet. 2021;12:633125. https://doi.org/10.3389/fgene.2021.633125. PMID: 33968129; PMCID: PMC8100685.
17. Mayer B, Kis Z, Kaján G, Frenyó LV, Hammarström L, Kacskovics I. The neonatal fc receptor (FcRn) is expressed in the bovine lung. Vet Immunol Immunopathol. 2004;98(1–2):85–9. https://doi.org/10.1016/j.vetimm.2003.10.010. PMID: 15127845.
18. Ellis JA, West KH, Waldner C, Rhodes C. Efficacy of a saponin-adjuvanted inactivated respiratory syncytial virus vaccine in calves. Can Vet J. 2005;46(2):155–62.
19. Steff AM, Monroe J, Friedrich K, Chandramouli S, Nguyen TL, Tian S, Vandepaer S, Toussaint JF, Carfi A. Pre-fusion RSV F strongly boosts pre-fusion specific neutralizing responses in cattle pre-exposed to bovine RSV. Nat Commun. 2017;8(1):1085. https://doi.org/10.1038/s41467-017-01092-4. PMID: 29057917; PMCID: PMC5651886. 1.
20. West K, Petrie L, Konoby C, Haines DM, Cortese V, Ellis JA. The efficacy of modified-live bovine respiratory syncytial virus vaccines in experimentally infected calves. Vaccine. 1999;18(9–10):907–19. https://doi.org/10.1016/s0264-410x(99)00324-2. PMID: 10580205.
21. Palmer MV, Wiarda J, Kanipe C, Thacker TC. Early pulmonary lesions in cattle infected via aerosolized Mycobacterium bovis. Vet Pathol. 2019;56(4):544–54. https://doi.org/10.1177/0300985819833454.
22. Chai J, Capik SF, Kegley B, Richeson JT, Powell JG, Zhao J. Bovine respiratory microbiota of feedlot cattle and its association with disease. Vet Res. 2022;53:4. https://doi.org/10.1186/s13567-021-01020-x.
23. Howe S, Kegley B, Powell J, Chen S, Zhao J. Effect of bovine respiratory disease on the respiratory microbiome: a meta-analysis. Front Cell Infect Microbiol. 2023;13:1223090. https://doi.org/10.3389/fcimb.2023.1223090. PMID: 37743862; PMCID: PMC10516580.
24. Murray GM, More SJ, Sammin D, et al. Pathogens, patterns of pneumonia, and epidemiologic risk factors associated with respiratory disease in recently weaned cattle in Ireland. J Vet Diagn Invest. 2017;29(1):20–34. https://doi.org/10.1177/1040638716674757.

Immunotherapies

13

Abstract

Immunotherapies are the fastest-growing area of novel therapeutics in medicine today. These treatments may be derived from the immune system itself or can be therapies that modulate the immune system to attempt better outcomes for the animal. Immunotherapies have been developed for disease treatment and prevention, dermatology, cancer, endocrine adjustments, allergy modification, and general immune system modulation (Thacker EL. Vet Clin North Am Small Anim Pract 40(3):473–483, 2010; Mueller RS et al. Allergy 73(10):1989–1999. https://doi.org/10.1111/all.13464, 2018; DeBoer DJ. Vet Dermatol 28(1):25–e6. https://doi.org/10.1111/vde.12416, 2017). Immunotherapies can either suppress or enhance immune responses depending on the outcome needed for a particular disease syndrome. While not all are used in cattle, immunotherapeutics have been used in bovine medicine for decades.

Keywords

Immunotherapy · Monoclonal antibody · Serum · Tetanus antitoxin · Polyclonal antibodies · Cytokines · Vaccination · Immunocastration · Somatostatin · Toll cell-like receptor · Immunogenomics · Immunogenetics

Key Concepts

- Immunotherapies are the fastest-growing area of new treatments in medicine today.
- Treatments may be derived from the immune system or used to stimulate the immune system.

J. Ellis, V. Cortese, *Practical Bovine Immunology*,
https://doi.org/10.1007/978-3-032-15031-8_13

- Areas utilizing immunotherapies include disease treatment and prevention, dermatology, cancer, endocrine modulation, allergy modification, and general immune system modulation [1–3].
- While not all are used in cattle, immunotherapeutics have been used in bovine medicine for decades.

What Is Immunotherapy?

Immunotherapy is defined as a treatment or prevention of disease by *activating, supporting, modulating, or suppressing* the immune system. Much of the human immunotherapy research focuses on cancer therapies. In veterinary medicine, immunotherapies are also available for infectious disease prevention and treatment, pain management, arthritis and dermatitis treatments, and modification of the endocrine system. Vaccination may be considered a form of immunotherapy in the broadest definition. Vaccines can be designed or have the ability through secondary effects, not only for prevention, but as a therapeutic strategy to treat diseases. These vaccines are routinely used in cattle and are covered in Chap. 13.

Immunotherapies that elicit or amplify an immune response are classified as *activation or modulation immunotherapies*, while immunotherapies that decrease or suppress are classified as *suppression immunotherapies*. Some immunotherapies do not directly impact the immune system but treat or prevent disease by indirectly stimulating the immune system [1].

What Immunotherapies Are Used in Cattle Today?

A. Multiple Antibody Treatment

The very first immunotherapy used in cattle was tetanus antitoxin. In the early 1900s, serum, derived from hyperimmunized horses and sheep, was collected and used, primarily as a treatment for tetanus [4, 5]. While the exact mechanisms at that time were not understood, the use of tetanus antitoxin from hyperimmunized horses is still used in calves today as a preventative and treatment.

As more was understood about the use of serum and antibodies, serum from cows was administered to calves with failure of passive transfer [4]. While it was recognized that the serum contained more than antibodies, the primary goal was to increase antibody levels, and serum transfusions progressed to serum from hyperimmunized cattle [4–6]. Hyperimmunization programs had three different immunotherapeutic applications beyond improving serum or colostrum. The first was the development of other polyclonal antibody preparations beyond tetanus antitoxin. Larger volume, more purified serum products, focusing on antibodies only, became commercially available [7, 8]. The second was the advent of colostral replacers and supplements. In both powdered and bolus form, these products are made from colostrum collected from well or hyper-immunized cows [9]. Finally, as a more affordable method of obtaining antibodies, eggs are injected with different pathogens, and egg-derived antibodies are harvested (primarily IgY) and used for the prevention of respiratory and gastrointestinal diseases in cattle.

B. Monoclonal Antibodies

The focus on antibody immunotherapy continued, but the cost of maintaining herds of animals and the chances of contaminated products drove research to develop laboratory-engineered antibodies. Monoclonal antibodies are identical immunoglobulins, generated from a single B-cell clone. These antibodies recognize unique epitopes, or binding sites, on a single antigen. Monoclonal antibodies are derived from a single B-cell clone and are usually expressed in a recombinant system (bacterial or murine) that expresses the desired antibody [10–13].

Some of the first monoclonal antibodies available for use in cattle were against the *E. coli* K99 pilus antigen [14]. Since monoclonal antibodies can be used for the prevention of disease, targeting of specific cells, blocking cytokines and hormones, and in immunodiagnostics, they are one of the fastest growing areas of immunotherapies and will continue to be developed for use in livestock production [10, 15].

C. Immunomodulating by Vaccination

The ability of vaccines, either as a primary or as a secondary benefit, to modulate or enhance the immune response generically has been utilized in cattle for decades. The best example is the use of Bacillus Calmette–Guérin (BCG) vaccine as part of a treatment regimen for ocular squamous cell carcinoma (cancer eye). The BCG vaccine is a potent stimulator of B and T cells and improves natural killer cell activity [16]. A secondary benefit of intranasal modified live herpesvirus vaccination is cytokine release, particularly several different interferons [17, 18]. Finally, as pointed out in Chap. 16, some adjuvants used in vaccines have immunomodulating effects.

D. Cytokine Immunotherapy

Cytokine and cytokine blocker therapies have great potential for treating a variety of diseases. As intercellular messengers, they control the immune response via signaling pathways in various types of leukocytes. Since many are pro-inflammatory, cytokine blockers may be useful in limiting inflammatory responses. Since cytokines have activity on many different cell types and tissues, serious adverse events associated with their use are a concern, and a correct dosage is critical. It has been difficult to show the clinical benefit of using these types of products [19–21]. The best examples of cytokine therapy assessed in cattle are bovine granulocyte colony-stimulating factor (Pegbovigrastim) and bovine interferon gamma. While both have shown great potential (primarily in immune response tests), individual variations in response have proven that it is difficult or impossible to optimize the immune system using a single chemical/synthetic inducer, and field trials did not show consistent benefits [21–23]. While these products may be used in the future, they are primarily used in cattle diagnostics and immune system research. Cytokine blockers are used in canine medicine for the treatment of allergic conditions.

E. Toll Cell-Like Receptor Agonists and Blockers

Toll cell-like receptor (TLR) agonists are used in veterinary medicine as adjuvants and immunostimulators [24–26]. Since each TLR responds to a specific pathogen-associated molecular pattern (PAMP), TLR agonists are PAMPs that are manufactured to stimulate specific TLRs. These products are usually in nanoparticles (NP-TLR agonists) [24–27].

One product utilizing this technology is currently available for use in cattle as an immunostimulator in stressed cattle [28–30]. TLR antagonists are being studied as a possible treatment for inflammatory diseases [31].

F. Immunoendocrinology

A relatively new immunotherapy area is the use of the immune system to impact physiologic functions such as sexual behavior, growth, feed efficiency, and milk production. Anti-gonadotrophin-releasing hormone vaccines were the first products in this category to be used in production medicine. These vaccines are used for immunocastration, estrus control, and immunologic spaying of feedlot heifers [32–34]. Variation in vaccination schedules can determine whether the outcome is permanent or temporary. These vaccines have also been used as treatment for some cancers and in conjunction with anti-luteinizing hormone-releasing hormone vaccines, studied as a contraceptive [35, 36]. For production medicine, the most exciting research involves anti-somatostatin vaccines. Shown to improve weight gain and feed efficiency, these products may also increase milk production and milk production efficiency [37–39].

G. Immunogenomics and Immunogenetics

While often used interchangeably, genetics focuses on the study of individual genes and their inheritance patterns, whereas genomics studies all the genes in an organism, including their interactions and variations. It involves analyzing the entire genome, which is the complete set of an organism's DNA, to determine the genetic basis of complex traits and diseases [40, 41].

While there are several thousand genes that are responsible for immune responses in cattle, research continues to determine which genes impact different immune responses and confer disease resistance. The goal is to breed or genetically engineer cattle for resistance to disease [42, 43]. Genomic testing and selection for specific disease resistance (mastitis, metritis, etc.) is already available and has an impact on lowering susceptibility to disease in beef and dairy herds utilizing the genomic tools [44–47].

H. Immune Cell Therapy

Immune cell therapy involves extracting and separating immune cells from the animal. The cells are modified or enhanced and given back to the individual to target and destroy cancer or fight off a specific disease. This method is still largely experimental in veterinary medicine, is very individualized in its approach, and is currently cost-prohibitive for use in production medicine.

Conclusion

The development and use of immunotherapies in cattle provides methods of enhancing and utilizing the immune system in unique ways. As more of the mysteries of the immune system are understood, this area of immunology will continue to expand as new products and treatment modalities become available and economically practical.

Your Case

You are called out by the owner of a 500-cow dairy in the upper Midwest to examine three fresh cows (under 10 days in milk) that are "off feed" and have a significant decrease in milk production. Upon examination, the cows are febrile (14.6–105.4 °F). There is a slight increase in respiratory rate and sounds, but otherwise, the examination is unremarkable. The owner explains that he began seeing cows with similar symptoms several months earlier. Most of the cows do not return to full production, and few have progressed into what he has diagnosed as pneumonia.

Cull rates have increased dramatically for cows in the first 60 days in milk due to poor lactation or pneumonia. You treat the cows symptomatically for the fever and prophylactically with a long-acting cephalosporin. ◄

Questions

1. What is your tentative diagnosis?
2. What do you do next?
3. Based on the results, what do you recommend?
4. Do you have any further suggestions if the recommendations do not work?

Additional Readings

1. Thacker EL. Immunomodulators, immunostimulants, and immunotherapies in small animal veterinary medicine. Vet Clin North Am Small Anim Pract. 2010;40(3):473–83.
2. Mueller RS, Jensen-Jarolim E, Roth-Walter F, Marti E, Janda J, Seida AA, DeBoer D. Allergen immunotherapy in people, dogs, cats and horses—differences, similarities and research needs. Allergy. 2018;73(10):1989–99. https://doi.org/10.1111/all.13464.
3. DeBoer DJ. The future of immunotherapy for canine atopic dermatitis: a review. Vet Dermatol. 2017;28(1):25–e6. https://doi.org/10.1111/vde.12416.
4. Silverstein AM. Emil von Behring: infectious disease, immunology, serum therapy: project MUSE, (review). Bull History Med. 2006;80:778–80.
5. Malaviya AN, Mehra NK. A fascinating story of the discovery & development of biologicals for use in clinical medicine. Indian J Med Res. 2018;148(3):263–78. https://doi.org/10.4103/ijmr.IJMR_1471_18. s
6. Chirgerwe M, Tyler JW. Serum IgG concentration after intravenous serum transfusion in a randomized clinical trial in dairy calves with inadequate transfer of colostral immunoglobulins. J Vet Internal Med. 2010;24:231–4.
7. Bresciani C, Sabbioni A, Ciampoli R, Bertocchi M, Saleri R, Cabassi CS. An innovative hyperimmune bovine plasma for prophylaxis and therapy of neonatal dairy calf diarrhea-a clinical trial. Large Anim Rev. 2016;22:115–9.
8. Selim SA, Holmberg CA, Cullor JS. Passive immunotherapy in neonatal calves. II. The efficacy of a J5 Escherichia coli hyperimmune plasma as immunotherapy in neonatal calves. Vaccine. 1995;13:1454–9.
9. Quigley JD, Strohbehn RE, Kost CJ, O'Brien MM. Formulation of colostrum supplements, colostrum replacers and acquisition of passive immunity in neonatal calves. J Dairy Sci. 2001;84(9):2059–65. https://doi.org/10.3168/jds.S0022-0302(01)74650-4. PMID: 11573786; PMCID: PMC7157919.
10. Van Der Lende T. Generation and applications of monoclonal antibodies for livestock production. Biotechnol Adv. 1994;12(1):71–87. ISSN 0734-9750. https://doi.org/10.1016/0734-9750(94)90291-7.
11. Malik B, Ghatol A. Understanding how monoclonal antibodies work. [Updated 2023 Jun 26]. In: StatPearls [Internet]. Treasure Island (FL): StatPearls Publishing; 2025. Available from: https://www.ncbi.nlm.nih.gov/books/NBK572118/.
12. Baker K, Eastwood TA, Garcia E, Lennon C, Mulvihill DP. Simple recombinant monoclonal antibody production from Escherichia coli. Open Biol. 2025;15(2):240229. https://doi.org/10.1098/rsob.240229. Epub 2025 Feb 19. PMID: 39965660; PMCID: PMC11835484.
13. Groves DJ, Tucker EM. The production and application of non-rodent monoclonal antibodies in veterinary science. Vet Immunol Immunopathol. 1989;23(1–2):1–14. https://doi.org/10.1016/0165-2427(89)90105-0. PMID: 2694587; PMCID: PMC7133.
14. Sherman DM, Acres SD, Sadowski PL, et al. Protection of calves against fatal enteric colibacillosis by orally administered Escherichia coli K99-specific monoclonal antibody. Infect Immun. 1983;42(2):653–8. https://doi.org/10.1128/iai.42.2.653-658.1983.
15. Wang J, Zhou X, Elazab ST, Huang J, Hsu WH. Current review of monoclonal antibody therapeutics in small animal medicine. Animals (Basel). 2025;15(4):472. https://doi.org/10.3390/ani15040472. PMID: 40002954; PMCID: PMC11852019.
16. Podarala V, Lakshmi MP, Rayadurgam Venkata SK, Devalam RP. Efficacy of BCG vaccine and Mitomycin C for the treatment of ocular squamous cell carcinoma in bovines. Res Vet Sci. 2020;133:48–52. ISSN 0034-5288. https://doi.org/10.1016/j.rvsc.2020.08.008.
17. Cortese VS, Woolums A, Hurley DJ, Berghaus R, Bernard JK, Short TH. Comparison of interferon and bovine herpesvirus-1-specific IgA levels in nasal secretions of dairy cattle administered an intranasal modified live viral vaccine prior to calving or on the day of calving. Vet Immunol Immunopath. 2017;187:35–41.

18. Woolums AR, Siger L, Johnson S, Gallo G, Conlon J. Rapid onset of protection following vaccination of calves with multivalent vaccines containing modified-live or modified-live and killed BHV-1 is associated with virus-specific interferon gamma production. Vaccine. 2003;21(11–12):1158–64. ISSN 0264-410X. https://doi.org/10.1016/S0264-410X(02)00560-1.
19. Lowenthal JW, O'Neil TE, David A, Strom G, Andrew ME. Cytokine therapy: a natural alternative for disease control. Vet Immunol Immunopathol. 1999;72(1–2):183–8. ISSN 0165-2427. https://doi.org/10.1016/S0165-2427(99)00131-2.
20. Donnelly RP, Young HA, Rosenberg AS. An overview of cytokines and cytokine antagonists as therapeutic agents. Ann N Y Acad Sci. 2009;1182:1–13. https://doi.org/10.1111/j.1749-6632.2009.05382.x. PMID: 20074270; PMCID: PMC6580416.
21. Scheerlinck JP, Yen HH. Veterinary applications of cytokines. Vet Immunol Immunopathol. 2005;108(1–2):17–22. https://doi.org/10.1016/j.vetimm.2005.08.001.
22. Ruiz R, Tedeschi LO, Sepúlveda A. Investigation of the effect of pegbovigrastim on some periparturient immune disorders and performance in Mexican dairy herds. J Dairy Sci. 2017;100(4):3305–17. ISSN 0022-0302. https://doi.org/10.3168/jds.2016-12003.
23. Ohmann HB, Lawman MJ, Babiuk LA. Bovine interferon: its biology and application in veterinary medicine. Antivir Res. 1987;7(4):187–210. https://doi.org/10.1016/0166-3542(87)90028-3. PMID: 2441661; PMCID: PMC7133961.
24. Parra FL, Morilla MJ, Romero EL. Toll-like receptor agonist-based nanomedicines as veterinary immunotherapies. Precis Nanomed. 2020;3(3):577–607.
25. Oboge H, Riitho V, Nyamai M, Omondi GP, Lacasta A, Githaka N, Nene V, Aboge G, Thumbi SM. Safety and efficacy of toll-like receptor agonists as therapeutic agents and vaccine adjuvants for infectious diseases in animals: a systematic review. Front Vet Sci. 2024;11:1428713. https://doi.org/10.3389/fvets.2024.1428713. PMID: 39355141; PMCID: PMC11442433.
26. Fitzgerald KA, Kagan JC. Toll-like receptors and the control of immunity. Cell. 2020;180(6):1044–66. https://doi.org/10.1016/j.cell.2020.02.041.
27. Mansilla F, Takagi M, Garcia-Castillo V, Aso H, Nader-Macias ME, Vignolo G, Kitazawa H, Villena J. Modulation of toll-like receptor-mediated innate immunity in bovine intestinal epithelial cells by lactic acid bacteria isolated from feedlot cattle. Benef Microbes. 2020;11(3):269–82. https://doi.org/10.3920/BM2019.0189. Epub 2020 May 4. PMID: 32363914.
28. Warshakoon HJ, Hood JD, Kimbrell MR, Malladi S, Wu WY, Shukla NM, Agnihotri G, Sil D, David SA. Potential adjuvantic properties of innate immune stimuli. Hum Vaccin. 2009;5(6):381–94. https://doi.org/10.4161/hv.5.6.8175. Epub 2009 Jun 16. PMID: 19270494.
29. Woolums AR, Karisch BB, Parish JA, Park J, Seo KS, Badial P, Olsen SC. Effect of a DNA-based immunostimulant on growth, performance, and expression of inflammatory and immune mediators in beef calves abruptly weaned and introduced to a complete ration. J Anim Sci. 2019;97(1):111–21. https://doi.org/10.1093/jas/sky392. PMID: 30329060; PMCID: PMC6313151.
30. Ilg T. Investigations on the molecular mode of action of the novel immunostimulator zelnate: activation of the cgas-STING pathway in mammalian cells. Mol Immunol. 2017;90:182–9. https://doi.org/10.1016/j.molimm.2017.07.013.
31. Hennessy E, Parker A, O'Neill L. Targeting Toll-like receptors: emerging therapeutics? Nat Rev Drug Discov. 2010;9:293–307. https://doi.org/10.1038/nrd3203.
32. Siel D, Huenchullán PR, Vidal S, Valdés A, Sáenz L. Improving beef cattle production: safety and effectiveness of new immunocastration vaccine. Animals Basel. 2024;14(17):2538. https://doi.org/10.3390/ani14172538. PMID: 39272323; PMCID: PMC11394353.695.
33. Geary TW, Grings EE, MacNeil MD, de Avila DM, Reeves JJ. Use of recombinant gonadotropin-releasing hormone antigens for immunosterilization of beef heifers. J Animal Sci. 2006;84(2):343–50. https://doi.org/10.2527/2006.842343x.
34. Herbert C, Trigg T. Applications of GnRH in the control and management of fertility in female animals. Anim Reprod Sci. 2005;88:141–53. https://doi.org/10.1016/j.anireprosci.2005.05.007.

35. Campal-Espinosa AC, Junco-Barranco JA, Fuentes-Aguilar F, Calzada-Aguilera L, Rivacoba-Betancourt A, Rodríguez-Bueno RH, Bover-Campal AC, Bover-Fuentes EE, González L, de Quesada L, Alvarez A, Garay-Pérez HE. Influence of humoral response against GnRH, generated by immunization with a therapeutic vaccine candidate on the evolution of patients with castration-sensitive prostate adenocarcinoma. Technol Cancer Res Treat. 2023;22:15330338231207318. https://doi.org/10.1177/15330338231207318. PMID: 37828833; PMCID: PMC10576932.
36. Thau R. Anti-LHRH and anti-pituitary gonadotropin vaccines: their development and clinical applications. Scand J Immunol Suppl. 1992;11:127–30. https://doi.org/10.1111/j.1365-3083.1992.tb01635.x. PMID: 1514027.
37. Chalupa W, Schneider PL. Bovine somatotropin: physiology, lactational responses and implications for the dairy industry. Prof Anim Sci. 1986;2(1):27–36. ISSN 1080-7446. https://doi.org/10.15232/S1080-7446(15)32418-9.
38. National Research Council (US) Committee on Technological Options to Improve the Nutritional Attributes of Animal Products. Designing foods: animal product options in the marketplace. Washington (DC): National Academies Press (US); 1988. Immunization of Beef Cattle Against Somatostatin. Available from: https://www.ncbi.nlm.nih.gov/books/NBK218172/.
39. Spencer GS. New approach to regulation of growth using immunization against somatostatin: discussion paper. J R Soc Med. 1984;77(6):496–500. https://doi.org/10.1177/014107688407700611. PMID: 6204049; PMCID: PMC1439815.
40. Meade KG. Advances in bovine immunology - new tools and new insights to tackle old foes. Front Immunol. 2015;6:71. https://doi.org/10.3389/fimmu.2015.00071. PMID: 25741343; PMCID: PMC4330913.
41. Garg AD. The dynamic interface of genetics and immunity: toward future horizons in health & disease. Genes Immun. 2023;24:155–8. https://doi.org/10.1038/s41435-023-00213-y.
42. Lewin HA. Disease resistance and immune response genes in cattle: strategies for their detection and evidence of their existence. J Dairy Sci. 1989;72(5):1334–48. https://doi.org/10.3168/jds.S0022-0302(89)79241-9. PMID: 2501367.
43. Mallard BA, Emam M, Paibomesai M, Thompson-Crispi K, Wagter-Lesperance L. Genetic selection of cattle for improved immunity and health. Jpn J Vet Res. 2015;63(Suppl 1):S37–44. PMID: 25872325.
44. Raszek MM, Guan l L, Plastow GS. Use of genomic tools to improve cattle health in the context of infectious diseases. Front Genet. 2016;7:30. https://doi.org/10.3389/fgene.2016.00030. PMID: 27014337; PMCID: PMC4780072.
45. Kasimanickam R, Ferreira JCP, Kastelic J, Kasimanickam V. Application of genomic selection in beef cattle disease prevention. Animals (Basel). 2025;15(2):277. https://doi.org/10.3390/ani15020277. PMID: 39858277; PMCID: PMC11759163.
46. Gutierrez-Reinoso MA, Aponte PM, Garcia-Herreros M. Genomic analysis, progress and future perspectives in dairy cattle selection: a review. Animals (Basel). 2021;11(3):599. https://doi.org/10.3390/ani11030599. PMID: 33668747; PMCID: PMC7996307.
47. Wiggans GR, Carrillo JA. Genomic selection in United States dairy cattle. Front Genet. 2022;13:994466. https://doi.org/10.3389/fgene.2022.994466. PMID: 36159997; PMCID: PMC9500184.

Bovine Vaccination

14

Abstract

Vaccination is one of the primary ways the immune system prevents or decreases the severity of common diseases of cattle. There are several different types of vaccines that are available for use in cattle. Continued research in basic immunology and innovative vaccine options will offer new options for vaccination programs in cattle, many of which start at the earliest stages of an animal's life. Specific knowledge of mechanisms, applications, timing, and vaccine platforms is needed to avoid adverse reactions.

Keywords

Vaccination · Modified live · Inactivated · Non-living vaccines · Prime boost Immunodominance · Adverse reactions · Endotoxin · Adjuvants

Key Concepts

- Vaccination is one of the primary ways the immune system can be used to prevent or decrease the severity of the disease.
- There are several different types of vaccines that are available for use in cattle.
- Newer studies continue to use science to develop vaccination programs.
- Vaccination programs build from the calf through adulthood. However, care must be exercised to avoid adverse reactions.

J. Ellis, V. Cortese, *Practical Bovine Immunology*,
https://doi.org/10.1007/978-3-032-15031-8_14

Why Are Cattle Routinely Vaccinated?

Vaccinations are an important aspect of cattle management used for *preventing disease*, improving overall herd health and performance, decreasing sickness and death loss, and improving reproductive efficiency by reducing infertility, embryonic and fetal deaths, and abortions [1]. Vaccines contain immunologically important components (antigens, usually protein, and more recently, mRNA encoding immunostimulatory proteins) or entire disease-causing agents, usually viral or bacterial, that have been modified to reduce disease-causing capability. They stimulate the immune system to create an immune response that is strong enough to moderate the severity or stop the disease from targeted pathogens [2]. Ideal vaccines prevent the infection, but these are more theoretical, and most are produced to reduce the disease potential of infectious agents.

To design a vaccination program for a group of cattle, several factors need to be considered:

1. *Challenge*—In the real world faced by most bovine practitioners, the level of disease challenge and degree of protection of animals under their care are in a continual state of fluctuation. The *level of protection* is different in every vaccinated animal due to biological variability. An overwhelming challenge can override immunity and lead to disease even in well-vaccinated animals [1–3]. Of course, susceptibility to the challenge organism is an important component of the disease process.
2. *Timing of Disease*—Due to common production practices, many cattle operations, whether involving beef or dairy cattle, will have consistent times when certain diseases occur. The timing of disease patterns may give some insight into stresses and disease exposures that are occurring in the management of a particular cattle operation. This type of information is helpful to determine the type and timing of vaccinations. Knowing when and under what circumstances a disease problem has historically occurred will allow vaccinations to be selected and scheduled to provide maximum immune responses.
3. *Vaccine Efficacy*—Vaccine efficacy can be extremely difficult to assess. Traditionally, serologic data showing pre-and post-vaccination titers has been equated to protection. For many diseases, there is a poor correlation between an antibody being measured and the protection generated by the vaccine in the animal [3–5]. Cell-mediated immune function tests have been added to show a more complete stimulation of the immune response after vaccination [6, 7]. Although this gives more information on the vaccine, it still does not answer the basic question of how well a vaccine really protects. The best measurement of vaccine efficacy is by well-designed challenge studies. There are many examples of well-designed studies with both viral and bacterial agents. However, studies need to be carefully reviewed, and outcomes in the control, challenged animals must be available. Most challenge studies are based on licensing efficacy trials by the vaccine manufacturer. These results, in controlled environments with controlled challenges, are designed to maximize results and are the basic definition of

vaccine efficacy [8, 9]. Field trials are even harder to assess but are valuable at answering the effectiveness (i.e., the efficacy in a particular situation and cost-effectiveness of a vaccine) [10, 11]. There are several good references on vaccine trial analysis available [10, 11]. Unfortunately, for many of our diseases, a challenge model is not well established or does not closely mimic the naturally occurring disease.

What Are the Different Technologies Utilized in Cattle Vaccines?

There are basically two broad categories of vaccines available today in veterinary medicine: *modified-live* and *non-living* (both viral and bacterial vaccines) [1–4, 12]. While different and emerging vaccine technologies have been developed, they still follow these two broad categories and will be discussed as the subtypes of the broad category into which they fit. Not all the newer subtypes of vaccines are available in cattle vaccines, but they will be included as a reference for the basis of future vaccines utilizing these technologies as they become available.

Modified Live Vaccines

A. *Modified live (attenuated) viral* vaccines contain living viral organisms that have been modified. They are usually collected from an infected animal and then grown in the laboratory in cultures of cells that it wouldn't normally grow in (e.g., fibroblasts) to change or attenuate the pathogen. For modified-live virus (MLV) viruses, each time the culture of the pathogen is repeated, it is called a *passage*. After several passages, the modified virus will begin to lose virulence factors since it cannot cause "disease" in these unnatural host cells. After several passages, it is administered back to the animal to see if it is still virulent. Once the pathogen can no longer cause "disease" in the target species, it is then tested to see if it can confer protection. The final vaccine is usually passed several times beyond the passage where virulence is no longer seen. This decreases the risk of reversion to a virulent pathogen. These vaccines require good quality control to decrease the risk of a contaminant entering the vaccine. When administered, modified live vaccines replicate in the animal and can stimulate immune responses similar to a natural infection by the "wild" virus.

   (a) *Temperature-sensitive virus* variants are modified-live viral vaccines in which the viruses undergo decreased replication at the body temperature of the animal being vaccinated. Temperature-sensitive vial vaccines are available for Bovine Viral Diarrhea virus, Bovine herpesvirus 1 virus, and Parainfluenza 3 virus.
   (b) *Vector*-based vaccines differ from most vaccines in that they do not contain the pathogen and all its antigens. Instead, they use a modified virus (the vector) to deliver genetic code for some of a pathogen's antigens. When the vector virus infects cells, the host cell makes large amounts of antigen from

this genetic code, which then triggers an immune response. Since the vector is modified-live, it is considered a modified-live vaccine even though the pathogen being vaccinated against is not.

(c) *Gene-deleted* modified live vaccines remove genes of an organism so that it becomes genetically altered. Deletion of the genes can include those that code for proteins associated with virulence and/or replication and growth *in vivo*. It is also possible to alter the expression of specific antigens so that a vaccine will induce an antibody response distinguishable from that caused by wild strains. Most of these vaccines are modified live mutants (temperature-sensitive) viral vaccines, but inactivated marker vaccines can also be similarly genetically engineered.

B. *Modified-live bacterial* vaccines are similar in that they have been modified or selected to decrease or remove virulence. This can be achieved by several different methods, including selecting strains that are avirulent, choosing media or harvest times that select or develop avirulent strains, and using gene deletion technology to limit or change growth characteristics.

C. *Inactivated* (killed, non-living vaccines)

Initially referred to as inactivated or killed vaccines, newer methods of providing non-living antigens (e.g., subunit elements, conjugated/recombinant antigens, or synthetic proteins) have expanded the definition beyond traditional inactivated vaccines. The major concern with the inactivation or development of newer non-living technologies is the potential loss of important epitopes. These vaccines may be less immunogenic than modified live vaccines because they are unable to grow and are less likely to stimulate all aspects of the immune system in an optimal fashion. As a result, vaccines that contain killed organisms or purified antigens may require multiple doses, and many also require the use of adjuvants to maximize their effectiveness. In cattle, inactivated vaccines have been developed against bacteria, viruses, exotoxins, fungi, and endotoxins. While virulence is not an issue with non-living vaccines, adverse reactions (local and systemic) are more commonly seen with non-living vaccines.

(a) Traditional *inactivated (killed)* vaccines are easier to develop than modified live vaccines since virulence after growth is not a problem. The same pathogen is isolated from a disease outbreak. The pathogen is grown and then chemically or physically killed. The inactivation is usually achieved by either adding a chemical to the pathogens or using ultraviolet rays. Most of these vaccines require at least two doses (primary and booster) to provide protection, and most utilize an adjuvant to increase the immune response to the antigens. Since many of the antigens in an inactivated vaccine may not be involved in providing a protective immune response, newer technologies tend to focus immune responses against just the antigens that have been identified to be involved in protective immune responses.

(b) *Subunit* vaccines were the first of the 'newer" technologies based on using just antigens involved in driving immune responses that were protective. Subunit vaccines are made from a piece of a pathogen, not the whole organism, limiting the immune response to just those antigens in the subunit vaccine. Subunit antigens can be made from pieces of the actual pathogen, manufactured synthetic protein, or recombinant expression.

(c) *Recombinant* antigen vaccines are subunit vaccines. The difference is that the antigen is made and expressed by a different organism by introducing the genetic sequence of the protein into a bacterium or yeast. The organism then makes that antigen, which can be harvested and made into a subunit vaccine.

(d) *DNA plasmid* vaccines are a type of *DNA vaccine* that uses small, circular pieces of DNA called *plasmids* to instruct cells in the body to produce a specific protein from a pathogen. After growth and purification, the DNA plasmids are ready for administration as a vaccine, using a variety of delivery methods, each designed to enhance the uptake of DNA by host cells. Vaccine proteins are then made by the host and therefore contain important posttranslational modifications. But like subunit vaccines, DNA vaccines must be adjuvanted.

(e) *Messenger RNA (mRNA)* vaccines are much like the DNA vaccines, but simpler and more directed. Once an mRNA vaccine is delivered, the mRNA signals the cell to manufacture the antigen [13]. An mRNA molecule enables efficient translation of a DNA genetic sequence, without transcription, by directing the production of antigenic proteins by the ribosomes in the cytoplasm of the cells.

Immunologically, an important advantage of (modified) live vaccines, as well as DNA plasmid and mRNA vaccines, is that they can essentially “fool” the body’s cells, making them “think” they are infected. This allows antigen presentation by both major histocompatabiliy complrx (MHC)-I and MHC-II pathways and the stimulation of broader antibody and cell mediated immune responses. Inactivated vaccines, including subunit vaccines, cannot do that without specific adjuvants and can only be processed and presented by the MHC-II pathway, somewhat limiting responses (antibody and CD4+ T cells; Chaps. 3 and 4).

Each company’s development and manufacture of vaccines is different; thus, the composition of the vaccine will vary dramatically among different manufacturers. Outlines of production are proprietary for each manufacturer; however, some information can be found in technical and marketing pieces. The variability in manufacturing may be seen in the following areas:

- Strain(s) chosen for the vaccine
- Number of passages chosen in the growth
- Growth medium or cell lines used for growth
- Number of viral or bacterial particles in the vaccine
- Harvest times
- Adjuvants used

Once the efficacy has been established, then the vaccine is put through a series of experiments to determine the minimum dose required to give adequate protection, called the minimum immunizing dose (MID). The vaccine will contain more than the MID when it is released for sale to ensure at least the MID in the vaccine at the expiration date found on the label. In effect, a vaccine's efficacy is not determined with the final product used by the veterinarian, but at a reduced level of immunogens from the amount contained in the final vaccine.

What Are Autogenous Vaccines?

Autogenous vaccines are a special class of vaccines that are custom vaccines since the isolate(s) used to make the autogenous product are from the herd of origin [14, 15]. Under normal circumstances, microorganisms from one herd should not be used to prepare an autogenous biologic for another herd. Autogenous vaccine manufacturing and requirements for their use are not regulated in many countries. Even when they are regulated, autogenous vaccines have limited or no efficacy data and minimal safety data. Autogenous products should be considered only when no commercially licensed product is available, or when commercially licensed products have not provided adequate protection against a particular pathogen.

What Is an Adjuvant?

An adjuvant is a compound that is added to vaccines (usually non-living) to increase or modulate the immune response to that vaccine [16]. An *immunologic adjuvant* is defined as any substance that acts to accelerate, prolong, or enhance antigen-specific immune responses when used in combination with specific vaccine antigens [17]. There are four primary classes of adjuvants based on their mode of action, and they can be comprised of organic and/or inorganic compounds.

1. *Depot adjuvants* protect the antigen and prolong the amount of time that an antigen is presented to the immune system. These adjuvants can act as a carrier molecule that entrap, adsorb, or aggregate antigens and release them slowly over a long period of time [16–20]. *Alum* (short for *aluminum salts*, such as aluminum hydroxide or aluminum phosphate) is considered a *depot adjuvant* and is commonly used in human and veterinary vaccines, for example, in some clostridial vaccines. Many depot types of adjuvants include an oil component [18, 19].
2. A second method in which adjuvants affect immune responses is by *improving antigen presentation* to the immune system [16–19]. The adjuvant may change the physical properties of the antigen. For example, it may increase the surface area of the antigen or form a polymer, thereby improving the presentation of the antigen to the immune system.
3. A third way that adjuvants work is by directly *enhancing or directing the immune response*. Compounds that do this can stimulate an immune response without an antigen being present and mostly function by causing the production of certain types of cytokines to potentiate the body's overall immune response. This is

often achieved by inclusion of molecules from foreign microbes pathogen-associated molecular patterns (PAMPs), or by causing some level of tissue damage-associated molecular patterns (DAMPs), either of which provides signals that can trigger innate responses that help to recruit and activate APCs and dendritic cells. This improves antigen presentation and stimulation of PRRs (e.g., Toll-like receptors) [16–20].

4. The final category includes adjuvants that combine different compounds to utilize several of the modes of action listed above in a single adjuvant system. For example, combination adjuvants like immune-stimulating complexes consisting of nanospheres made of QS-21, cholesterol, and phospholipids both enhance antigen presentation and have an immunomodulatory effect [16–19].

Do All Cattle Have a Protective Immune Response Following Vaccination?

When a population is exposed to a new pathogen, there is a *bell-shaped curve of susceptibility* (Fig. 14.1) [21]. While most animals are likely to get some degree of disease, there are some that are innately immune. Vaccination moves the population to a higher percentage that is protected (Fig. 14.2). Administration of a vaccine does not always provide protection. True non-responders to vaccination are rare and are usually genetic in nature [22]. However, poor responders are common due to many factors that influence the immune response to vaccination. These factors include stress, vitamin and mineral balance, poor nutrition, previous vaccination, colostral antibody levels in the newborn calf, vaccine handling and storage, and overall health of the animal being vaccinated [1–4, 21, 22]. Even under ideal conditions (licensing efficacy trials), no vaccine is 100% efficacious. Efficacy is usually lower in effectiveness trials and will vary by the antigen, a particular vaccine, the protection

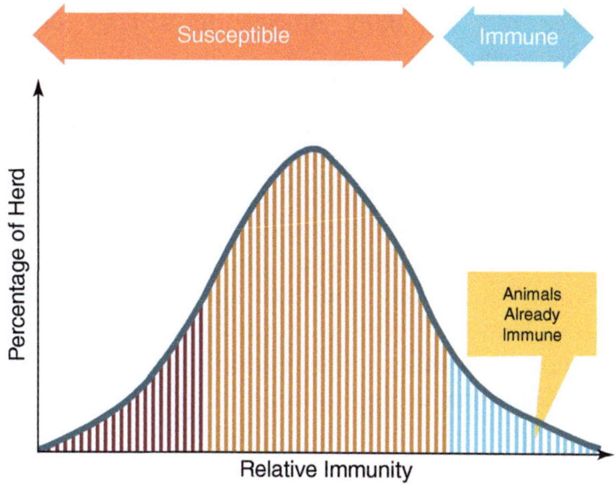

Fig. 14.1 Susceptibility curve of a naïve cattle population

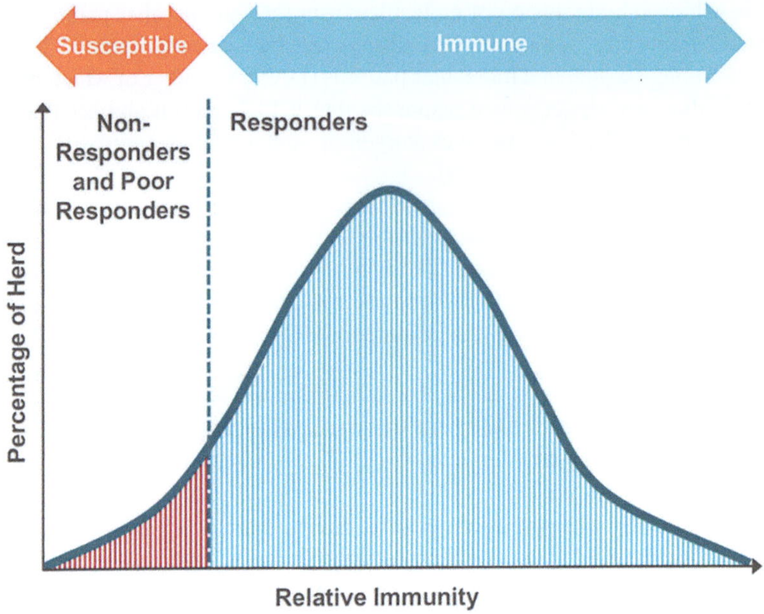

Fig. 14.2 Susceptibility curve of a cattle population after vaccination

desired (i.e., reproductive, in young animals, etc.), and the factors listed above. The goal of vaccination is to limit or prevent disease when an exposure (infection) occurs. Since much of the immune system responds after an infection has begun, the concept of "sterile" immunity, in which no pathogen can replicate or be detected after an exposure, is unrealistic. This can confuse the interpretation of diagnostic tests in which an infectious agent is found. The term sterilizing immunity may be misused to mean the absence of any clinical signs, which is complete protection [23].

The lack of 100% efficacy in a large population has two important ramifications.

1. Vaccination is to confer *herd immunity*, rather than individual immunity [22]. If a large enough percentage of the population is vaccinated, the dynamics of a particular pathogen's spread can be changed. The percentage required to be immune (naturally or following vaccination) to change a disease's transmission will vary by the pathogen.
2. Many studies have indicated that even with vaccines that have a single dose requirement, to provide protection on a herd basis, including at least two doses and/or shortening vaccine intervals will improve overall herd health. This is particularly true in high-challenge situations [23–25].

How Do Maternal Antibodies Impact Vaccination?

One of the issues common to both human and veterinary neonatology is the double-edged sword of *maternal antibodies (MAbs)*. Regardless of whether they are obtained across the placenta, as in humans and mice, or through timely ingestion of colostrum, as in domestic species, such as cattle, an adequate concentration of MAb assists in averting serious disease and sustaining life. Currently, in cattle, a total serum total protein (TP) of >6.2 g/dL and serum IgG of >25 g/L would be considered "excellent," whereas <5.1 g/dL TP and <10.0 gL would be considered "poor" [26]. Good passive transfer is a primary predictor of calf health [27].

On the other side of the sword, it is long and well established in both human [28] and veterinary medicine [29] that MAb, consistent with good passive transfer, can significantly interfere with the induction of some immune responses by injectable vaccines [28, 29]. Most studies have shown that animals vaccinated with injectable vaccines may not have increased antibody levels if there are high levels of *MAb* to that antigen [1–4]. In cattle, this inhibitory phenomenon was clearly demonstrated in robust challenge models of some important calfhood pathogens, including bovine viral diarrhea virus (BVDV) [30] and bovine respiratory syncytial virus (BRSV) [31]. In those models, calves, with good passive immunity, that were vaccinated parenterally with representative combination modified-live vaccines and then challenged months later after MAb had decayed, developed severe disease similar to placebo-vaccinated controls. Demonstrating interference by MAb also depends on what immune responses are measured. Thus, some studies have shown stimulation of both B and T cell memory responses in animals vaccinated when they have high levels of *MAb*, even if serum antibody levels do not change following vaccinated [33–38]. For example, sero-positive calves vaccinated at a young age with modified live BHV-1, PI3, or BRSV were shown to have higher antibody responses on revaccination compared to control calves that received a primary immunization at the same time [33, 37]. These young re-vaccinates did not have increased antibody responses after the first vaccination in the presence of high *MAb*. Cell-mediated (memory T cell) immune responses, as indicated by antigen-specific T cell blastogenesis, have also been demonstrated at weaning when neonatal calves were vaccinated in the face of maternal antibody [29] with attenuated BRSV and BHV-1 vaccines. Another factor that can contribute to the efficacy of vaccinating when maternal antibodies are present is vaccine formulation, notably the form of an antigen [33] and inclusion of a potent adjuvant [32, 38]. Nevertheless, it is important to remember that interference with immunization by injectable vaccines is not an "all-or-none" phenomenon, but rather a sliding scale, at least somewhat dependent on the concentration of MAbs [31, 32]. This is one reason why it is usually recommended that young animals, including calves, dogs, and humans, receive more than a single dose of injectable vaccine early in life because it is difficult to predict when MAb concentrations have decayed enough to allow optimal immunization.

Since young calf vaccination is a routine part of most cattle vaccination programs, when vaccination with conventional injectable vaccines is the only option in calves <3 months old, then, in most cases, that will be better than no vaccine at all.

However, owners should be informed as to the limitations of that approach. A better alternative when vaccinating young seropositive calves is to use mucosal (intranasal) delivery. The efficacy of this approach in stimulating protective clinical immunity in calves with maternal antibodies has been clearly documented in challenge models for BRSV [39] and BHV-1 [40]. The immunological reason for the apparent lack of interference by MAb using this route of administration is not "overriding" *MAbs*, but rather, avoiding them, since there is little, potentially neutralizing, (maternal) IgG (or the calf's own immune exclusionary IgA) in the nasal cavity of a normal healthy calf.

How Does Stress Affect an Immune Response?

Stress can impact the systemic immune system of all ages of cattle. There are several factors that can affect the immune system. The birthing process has a dramatic impact on the newborn's immune system due to corticosteroid release. Furthermore, the newborn has an increased number of suppressor T cells [2–4]. These factors and others decrease systemic immune responses for the first week of life. Procedures such as castrations, dehorning, weaning, and movement need to be considered as stresses in cattle, and all have the potential to decrease immune system function temporarily [41–50]. The impact of calving on post-partum stress and immune responses in dairy cattle has been extensively studied [50–54]. This stress had an impact on viral vaccines administered within 30 days post-calving [55]. Based on these studies, systemic vaccinations during high-stress times should be avoided if possible. However, new studies have indicated that, during periods of physiologic stress, the mucosal immune systems may not be compromised, and locally applied vaccines may be beneficial [56–60].

What Is the Importance of "Booster Shots"?

It is important to follow the label directions for administering vaccines. Inactivated vaccines and some modified-live vaccines require *a booster* before protection is complete [1, 2, 4]. The first time a vaccine requiring a booster is administered, the primary response occurs. This is short-lived and provides limited protection that is easy to overwhelm. The response seen after a booster vaccination is called the secondary, memory, or anamnestic response. If the booster is given too early, the anamnestic response does not occur, and if too much time elapses before the booster is given, it acts as an initial dose, not as a booster [1, 2, 4, 61]. The specific vaccine label will contain information on booster administration timing and should be followed. Research with specific vaccines occasionally indicates a broader window for boostering [61–63]. With most modified live vaccines, the replication of the (live) constituents from the primary vaccination also stimulates the secondary response without needing a booster [1, 2, 4].

What Causes Adverse Reactions to Vaccination?

Adverse reactions are a potential risk with any vaccination. These reactions fall into four primary categories [1, 2, 4, 64–71]:

1. *Type 1 hypersensitivity* (acute anaphylaxis) is mediated by IgE and the release of granules from basophils and mast cells to cause an immediate hypersensitivity. This reaction is seen within minutes of vaccination and often begins with shaking or sweating and swelling of extremities or the face. If treated immediately, the majority of these animals will respond to epinephrine [1, 2, 64, 65, 71].
2. *Type 2 hypersensitivity* is mediated by an antibody–antigen complex attaching to complement and the ensuing activation of the complement cascade [2]. The resultant reaction may occur locally or systemically. The reaction may be delayed as the complexes form, and the cascade begins, and subsequently, by-products begin to exert their effects. The signs are similar to immediate hypersensitivity, and treatment is epinephrine.
3. *Innate immune responses*: One of the more common reactions seen in cattle has been associated with endotoxin and other bacterial components found in most Gram-negative vaccines [66–71]. These components of Gram-negative vaccines are PAMPs that can cause the release of large amounts of proinflammatory cytokines by the innate immune system [68, 69, 71]. Currently, there are no requirements for monitoring or reporting the amount of endotoxin found in cattle vaccines, and the level of endotoxin may vary dramatically between vaccines and serials of the same vaccine [72]. The potency of endotoxin varies among different Gram-negative bacteria [66, 69, 70]. Vaccine storage and handling can also increase the endotoxin levels in a vaccine [70]. There is also a genetic predisposition in some animals that increases the risk and severity of reactions to these components and can be seen following administration of any Gram-negative bacterin [74–78]. Furthermore, the likelihood and severity of these reactions may increase with increased ambient temperature [70, 73, 74] and some nutritional deficiencies (see Chap. 9). The signs seen vary depending on the farm's or individual's sensitivity to Gram-negative bacterial components. The number or severity of the Gram-negative fractions in the vaccination program administered simultaneously is also instrumental in causing these reactions. These adverse reactions include:

   (a) Anorexia, temperature elevations, lethargy and transient decreases in milk production and weight gain/feed efficiency
   (b) Early embryonic deaths
   (c) Abortions
   (d) Gram-negative bacterial (endotoxic) shock, requiring fluxinin or keprofen, steroids, antihistamines, and fluids, that can lead to death

4. *Local reactions* can vary in size and can be granulomas or sterile abscesses. The lesions are usually caused by the adjuvant(s) used in the vaccine, and there can be some involvement of innate immune responses [70, 71, 76–81]. While heat,

pain, and swelling are commonly seen at the injection site, most of these local reactions will resolve over time, although there may be blemishes or scar tissue following intramuscular administration [81]. Depending on the site of vaccination, these local reactions can occasionally cause lameness and severe damage [78]. In partially used bottles of vaccine, bacterial contamination is a possibility, and after administration, abscesses may occur [70, 71].

Newer Vaccination Strategies

Heterologous Prime-Boost Programs

One strategy now commonly used in bovine vaccination programs is called the "*heterologous prime-boost*" protocol. This involves priming the immune system to a target antigen delivered by one vector, route, or mechanism, and then selectively boosting this immunity by re-administering the antigen in the context of a second and distinct method, either a different form of the antigen or a different route of administration [82–84]. For example, priming with an intranasal vaccine and boosting with an injectable vaccine have been used to examine responses to BHV-1 [85], BRSV [86], BVDV [87], bovine coronavirus [88], BoPIV-3 [89]. This is different from traditional programs in which the antigen is boostered with the same vaccine given by the same route.

Many studies have highlighted the power of prime-boost strategies to broaden and lengthen immune responses.

Heterologous prime boost studies have been investigated with:

(a) Different routes of administration [33, 85–94]
(b) Different antigen presentations (i.e., modified live and vector vaccines) [95, 96]
(c) Modified live and inactivated vaccines [97–99]
(d) Different adjuvants, inactivation techniques, or components of non-living vaccines [99–102]

Heterologous prime boost programs do not always provide better immune responses or protection [94, 102, 103]. The sequence of the vaccines [85, 91], as well as the type of booster vaccine after the priming dose [86–90], may also be an important factor in the success of a heterologous prime boost program. Thus, research must be done with each pair of vaccines to determine if a heterologous prime-boost program can be utilized against a particular pathogen.

What Is Immunodominance?

The terms *dominant antigens* and *immunodominance* have been used interchangeably to describe a unique phenomenon of the immune system. The term immunodominance has become the accepted term in human immunology [104].

Immunodominance is defined as the process whereby immune expression or recognition of one epitope or antigen influences (usually suppressing or blocking) the recognition of a second distinct epitope or antigen [104–107]. Most studies have focused on the occurrence of immunodominance in immune responses to the multitude of epitopes within a specific antigen (virus or bacteria) [104–107]. On any bacteria or virus, only 0.2% of the possible epitopes elicit any measurable immune response [104]. These are termed immunodominant epitopes, and they have been shown to block immune responses to other epitopes called subdominant epitopes [104–107]. These basic concepts have been extended to interactions between concurrent administration of different vaccines. The majority of immunodominance studies in veterinary medicine have focused on the impact on antibody production. However, immunodominance can affect T and B cells as well [105–110]. Thus, there are several mechanisms by which immunodominance can occur [104, 108, 109].

Immunodominance between antigens in a multi-antigen vaccination program has been shown in several studies [63, 111–114]. Of particular importance is the interaction documented between BHV-1 vaccines and bacterins concurrently administered to naive cattle. Identified as one of the strongest immunodominant viruses in human immunology [115], herpesviruses are also immunodominant viruses in cattle. Several studies have demonstrated that systemic vaccination with a bovine herpesvirus 1 (infectious bovine rhinotracheitis virus, BHV-1) vaccine decreased or blocked the response to co-administered *Mannheimia haemolytica* vaccines if the cattle had not been previously vaccinated with BHV-1 [111, 112]. Some interference with Clostridial vaccination was also seen when concurrently administered with systemic BHV-1 vaccines [63].

These studies have compared the serologic responses to *M. hemolytica* bacterins with co-administration of attenuated BHV-1, and no *Mannheimia* challenges were performed. However, it is well accepted that antibodies against *M. hemolytica* are protective, and serum antibody titers, particularly against leukotoxin, correlate with protection against *M. hemolytica* challenge. When the vaccines were given to animals previously vaccinated, and/or the BHV-1 vaccine was administered via a different route (intranasal); depression of the *M. hemolytica* vaccine response was not seen [33]. This should be considered when designing vaccination programs aimed at decreasing bovine respiratory disease.

How Do You Design a Vaccination Program?

Designing a vaccination program requires a good history of the individual farm as well as a basic understanding of the immune system. The vaccines chosen should have good solid efficacy studies (as well as effectiveness and efficiency studies if possible) to ensure that the product can fulfill the needs of the farm or ranch. The establishment of good baseline immunity in the replacement heifers and the foundation vaccination program in the cows can have dramatic effects on the health and profitability of the herd and needs to be well planned.

While it is true that vaccination programs in cattle are generally customized to a particular facility, there are basic guidelines that serve as a beginning point for designing a vaccination program.

1. A history of the facility, including type (dairy, feedlot, etc.), typical handling times of the cattle, lifecycle of the cattle on the facility, history of disease issues, and other pertinent management in place (i.e., complete artificial insemination program)
   (a) In concert with this information, the information on the vaccines being considered needs to be included in the program design. These include duration of immunity, safety issues, label claims, and recommendations for booster administration.
2. Start with diseases that are easily transmissible and/or can have a significant economic impact. Generally, these include bovine viral diarrhea virus, bovine herpesevirus-1, and bovine respiratory syncytial virus. In parts of the world where foot and mouth disease is present, due to its impact on risk and severity of disease by other pathogens, this is usually the first virus to evaluate in the vaccination program.
3. Include diseases from which there is a high mortality rate, exposure risk is high, and/or it is necessary to prevent specific syndromes (i.e., abortion). These would include vaccinations against Clostridial and Leptospiral diseases, and in the dairy core vaccination program, endotoxin vaccines would be included here.
4. All breeding replacement animals should receive two MLV viral vaccinations against BVDV, BHV-1, and BRSV before entering the breeding program.
5. All vaccines used in breeding animals and animals intended for breeding purposes should have studies and/or labels indicating that they provide protection against the reproductive forms of the various components.
6. If vaccinating animals at a time in which *MAb* may be present, then studies and/or labels should indicate that they may provide protection in the face of *MAb*.
7. Final vaccines included in the program are usually for herd-specific problems and may include respiratory, gastrointestinal, and other pathogens.
8. Limit the number of bacterial vaccines (particularly Gram-negative vaccines) administered on the same day.
9. Try to avoid co-administration of the initial BHV-1 vaccination with bacterins.

A good starting reference for designing vaccination programs for cattle is in the AABP guidelines for vaccination [116]. Management decisions may be made that do not maximize the potential of the chosen product, and realistic expectations of all products should be well explained to the producer before they are used. The owner should be involved in the vaccine decision-making process, and all the information on the product should be shared.

Your Case

History

A 2000-cow Holstein dairy located in Torreón, Mexico. The dairy raises all of its calves and currently keeps all its heifers for replacements. The dairy is on a comprehensive vaccination program, which has been recently updated. The herd uses artificial insemination with a timed artificial insemination program exclusively on the cows; however, bull breeding is used on the heifers.

Vaccination History

Newborn calves are administered an intranasal vaccine (MLV BRSV, BoPIV-3, and BHV-1). A second dose is administered at 8 weeks of age with an MLV BVDV vaccine administered subcutaneously. At 4 months of age, a modified-live five-way viral vaccine with *Mannheimia hemolytica* vaccine is injected subcutaneously. At a year of age (pre-breeding), replacement heifers are vaccinated with a modified live five-way viral vaccine and five-way leptospirosis vaccine, RB 51 *Brucella abortus* vaccine, and a seven-way Clostridial vaccine. At pregnancy confirmation, a seven-way Clostridial and a five-way leptospirosis vaccine are administered.

Cows are vaccinated pre-breeding with a modified live five-way viral vaccine and five-way leptospirosis vaccine; at confirmed pregnancy, a five-way leptospirosis vaccine is given. At cessation of milking, the cows are administered a core J5 *E. coli* vaccine and a scours vaccine containing rotavirus, coronavirus, and K99 *E. coli* antigens.

In August, a group of 55 pre-breeding heifers were vaccinated in the middle of the afternoon. The ambient temperature was 35.5 °C (96 °F), and the humidity was 80%. The heifers were vaccinated with a modified live BHV-1, BPI3, BRSV, and BVDV (types 1 and 2) vaccine and five-way leptospirosis vaccine, RB 51 *B. abortus* vaccine, and a seven-way Clostridial vaccine as per the vaccination protocol. However, a *M. hemolytica* vaccine was added due to an increase in pneumonia in yearlings.

Problem

At 7:00 am the following morning, 12 heifers were found dead in the pen, and nine heifers were found recumbent and unable to rise. The heifers exhibited labored breathing with increased respiratory and heart rates. Temperatures were within normal ranges. Some animals had foam in their oral cavities and increased salivation.

Questions

1. What are your three primary rule-outs for this problem?
2. How can you differentiate between your suspected causes of death and sickness?
3. Are there any underlying issues to be explored in the case?
4. What treatments, if any, can you do for the remaining heifers?
5. What advice would you give the dairy to avoid the same problem in the future?

Additional Readings

1. Cortese VS. Use of biologics in prevention of infectious disease: bovine vaccines and herd vaccination program. In: Smith BP, Van Metre DC, Pusterla N, editors. Large animal internal medicine. 6th ed. CV Mosby Co.; 2020. p. 1635–41. ISBN 9780323554459. https://doi.org/10.1016/B978-0-323-55445-9.00048-3.
2. Tizard I. General principles of vaccination and vaccines. In: Veterinary Immunology, an introduction. 4th ed. Philadelphia: WB Saunders Co.; 1992. p. 261–4.
3. Blecha F. New approaches to increasing immunity in food animals. Vet Med. 1990.
4. Duffus WPH. Immunoprophylaxis. In: REW H, Gorman NT, editors. Veterinary clinical immunology. Philadelphia: W. B. Saunders; 1989. p. 205–11.
5. Kaeberle M. The elements of immunity. Large animal veterinarian. 1991.
6. Abbas AK, Lichtman AH, Pober JS. Antigen presentation and T-cell recognition and Molecular basis of T cell antigen recognition and activation. In: Cellular and molecular immunology. Philadelphia: WB Saunders Co; 1991. p. 115–68.
7. Hoffman M. Determining what immune cells. Res News. 1992;255:531–4.
8. Lau CS, Aw TC. Considerations in understanding vaccine effectiveness. Vaccines (Basel). 2022;11(1):20. https://doi.org/10.3390/vaccines11010020. PMID: 36679865; PMCID: PMC9864852.
9. Brennan OC, Moore JE, Moore PJA, Millar BC. Vaccination terminology: a revised glossary of key terms including lay person's definitions. J Clin Pharm Ther. 2022;47(3):369–82. https://doi.org/10.1111/jcpt.13516. Epub 2021 Aug 31. PMID: 34463972; PMCID: PMC8656271.
10. Ribble C. Assessing vaccine efficacy. Can Vet J. 1990;31.
11. Meinert CL. Clinical trials; design, conduct and analysis. New York: Oxford University Press; 1986. p. 3–18.
12. Aida V, Pliasas VC, Neasham PJ, North JF, McWhorter KL, Glover SR, Kyriakis CS. Novel vaccine technologies in veterinary medicine: a herald to human medicine vaccines. Front Vet Sci. 2021;8:654289. https://doi.org/10.3389/fvets.2021.654289. PMID: 33937377; PMCID: PMC8083957.
13. Gote V, Bolla PK, Kommineni N, Butreddy A, Nukala PK, Palakurthi SS, Khan W. A Comprehensive Review of mRNA Vaccines. Int J Mol Sci. 2023;24(3):2700. https://doi.org/10.3390/ijms24032700. PMID: 36769023; PMCID: PMC9917162.
14. United States Department of Agriculture, Marketing and Regulatory Programs, Animal and Plant Health Inspection Service, Veterinary Services. 113.113 Autogenous biologics. 9CFR (code of federal regulations) 113.113 Updated Apr. 21, 2010. https://www.ecfr.gov/current/title-9/section-113.113.
15. United States Department of Agriculture, Marketing and Regulatory Programs, Animal and Plant Health Inspection Service, Veterinary Services. Guidelines for Autogenous Biologics VS Memorandum (VSM) 800.69. updated Nov 2021;1–10.
16. Zhao T, Cai Y, Jiang YHX, Wei Y, Yu Y, Tian X. Vaccine adjuvants: mechanisms and platforms. Sig Transduct Target Ther. 2023;8(1):283. https://doi.org/10.1038/s41392-023-01557-7AU.
17. Sasaki S, Okuda K. The use of conventional immunologic adjuvants in DNA vaccine preparations. In: Lowrie DB, Whalen RG, editors. DNA vaccines: methods and protocols. Methods in molecular medicine, vol. 29. Humana Press; 2000. p. 241–50. https://doi.org/10.1385/1-59259-688-6:241. ISBN 978-0896035805.
18. Wu Z, Liu K. Overview of vaccine adjuvants. Med Drug Disc. 2021;11:100103. ISSN 2590-0986. https://doi.org/10.1016/j.medidd.2021.100103.
19. Facciolà A, Visalli G, Laganà A, Di Pietro A. An overview of vaccine adjuvants: current evidence and future perspectives. Vaccines (Basel). 2022;10(5):819. https://doi.org/10.3390/vaccines10050819. PMID: 35632575; PMCID: PMC9147349.
20. Tizard IR. Adjuvants and adjuvanticity. Vaccines for Veterinarians. 2021:75–86.e1. https://doi.org/10.1016/B978-0-323-68299-2.00016-2. Epub 2020 Jul 10. PMCID: PMC7348637.

21. Vakili ME, Mashhadi N, Ataollahi MR, Meri S, Kabelitz D, Kalantar K. Hepatitis B vaccine responders show higher frequencies of CD8+ effector memory and central memory T cells compared to non-responders. Scand J Immunol. 2024;100(5):e13402. https://doi.org/10.1111/sji.13402. Epub 2024 Aug 27.
22. Wichgers Schreur PJ, Kant J, van Keulen L, Moormann RJ, Kortekaas J. Four-segmented Rift Valley fever virus induces sterile immunity in sheep after a single vaccination. Vaccine. 2015;33(12):1459–64. https://doi.org/10.1016/j.vaccine.2015.01.077. Epub 2015 Feb 7.
23. Rodning SP, Marley MS, Zhang Y, Eason AB, Nunley CL, Walz PH, Riddell KP, Galik PK, Brodersen BW, Givens MD. Comparison of three commercial vaccines for preventing persistent infection with bovine viral diarrhea virus. Theriogenology. 2010;73(8):1154–63. https://doi.org/10.1016/j.theriogenology.2010.01.017. Epub 2010 Feb 23.
24. Newcomer BW, Walz PH, Givens MD, Wilson AE. Efficacy of bovine viral diarrhea virus vaccination to prevent reproductive disease: a meta-analysis. Theriogenology. 2015;83(3):360–5. ISSN 0093-691X. https://doi.org/10.1016/j.theriogenology.2014.09.028.
25. Newcomer BW, Cofield LG, Walz PH, Givens MD. Prevention of abortion in cattle following vaccination against bovine herpesvirus 1: a meta-analysis. Prev Vet Med. 2017;138:1–8. https://doi.org/10.1016/j.prevetmed.2017.01.005. Epub 2017 Jan 6. PMID: 28237224.
26. Lombard JE, Urie N, Garry F, Godden S, et al. Consensus recommendations on calf- and herd-level passive immunity in dairy calves in the United States. J Dairy Sci. 2020;103:7611–24.
27. Sutter F, Venjakob PL, Heuwieser W, Borchardt S. Association between transfer of passive immunity, health, and performance of female dairy calves from birth to weaning. J Dairy Sci. 2023;105:7043–55. https://doi.org/10.3168/jds.2022-22448.
28. Edwards KM. Maternal antibodies and infant immune responses to vaccines. Vaccine. 2015;47:6469–72. https://doi.org/10.1016/j.vaccine.2015.07.085.
29. Chappuis G. Neonatal immunity and immunization in early age: lessons from veterinary medicine. Vaccine. 1998;16:1468–72.
30. Ellis J, West K, Cortese V, Konoby C, Weigel D. Effect of maternal antibodies on induction and persistence of vaccine-induced immune responses against bovine viral diarrhea virus type II in young calves. JAVMA. 2001;219:351–6.
31. Ellis J, Gow S, Bolton M, Burdett W, Nordstrom S. Inhibition of priming for bovine respiratory syncytial virus-specific protective immune responses following parenteral vaccination of passively immune calves. Can Vet J. 2014;55(12):1180–5. PMID: 25477547; PMCID: PMC4231808.
32. Kolb EA, Buterbaugh RE, Rinehart CL, et al. Protection against bovine respiratory syncytial virus in calves vaccinated with adjuvanted modified-live vaccine administered in the face of maternal antibody. Vaccine. 2020;38:298–308. https://doi.org/10.1016/j.vaccine.2019.10.015.
33. Parker WL, Galyean ML, Winder JA, Cravens RL. Effects of vaccination at branding on serum antibody titers to viral agents of bovine respiratory disease (BRD) in newly weaned New Mexico calves. Proceedings, Western Section, American Society of Animal Science, AS 44, 1993.
34. Kimman TG, Westenbrink F, Straver PJ. Priming for local and systematic antibody memory responses to bovine respiratory syncytial virus: effect of amount of virus, viral replication, route of administration and maternal antibodies. Vet Immunol Immunopath. 1989;22:145–60.
35. Pyo HM, Hlasny M, Zhou Y. Influence of maternally-derived antibodies on live attenuated influenza vaccine efficacy in pigs. Vaccine. 2015;33(31):3667–72. https://doi.org/10.1016/j.vaccine.2015.06.044. Epub 2015 Jun 16. PMID: 26092308.
36. Ellis JA, Hassard LE, Cortese VS, Morley PS. Effects of perinatal vaccination on humoral and cellular immune responses in cows and young calves. JAVMA. 1996;208(3):393–9.
37. Stokka GL, Neville B, Seeger JT, Cortese VS, Gaspers JJ. Serological effect of two concurrent IBRV, BVDV, BRSV, PI3V, and Mannheimia haemolytica vaccination protocols and time interval between the first and second dose on the subsequent serological response to the BRSV and M. haemolytica fractions in suckling beef calves. Bov Pract. 2016;50(1):21–7.

38. Riffault S, Hägglund S, Guzman E, et al. A single shot pre-fusion-stabilized bovine RSV F vaccine is safe and effective in newborn calves with maternally derived antibodies. Vaccines (Basel). 2020;8(2):231. https://doi.org/10.3390/vaccines8020231. PMID: 32443437; PMCID: PMC7349975.
39. Ellis JA, Gow SP, Mahan S, Leyh R. Duration of immunity to experimental infection with bovine respiratory syncytial virus following intranasal vaccination of young passively immune calves. J Am Vet Med Assoc. 2013;243(11):1602–8. https://doi.org/10.2460/javma.243.11.1602. PMID: 24261811.
40. Mahan SM, Sobecki B, Johnson J, et al. Efficacy of intranasal vaccination with a multivalent vaccine containing temperature-sensitive modified-live bovine herpesvirus type 1 for protection of seronegative and seropositive calves against respiratory disease. JAVMA. 2016;248:1280–6.
41. Zavy MT, Juniewicsz PE, Phillips WA, VonTungeln DL. Effect of initial restraint, weaning, and transport stress on baseline and ACTH-stimulated cortisol responses in beef calves on different genotypes. Am J Vet Res. 1992;53(4):551–8.
42. Sconberg S, Nockels CF, Bennett BW, Bruyninckx W, Blancquaert AB. Effects of shipping, handling, adrenocorticotropic hormone, and epinephrine on a-tocopherol content of bovine blood. Am J Vet Res. 1993;54(8):1287–94.
43. VonTungeln DL. The effects of stress on the immunology of the stocker calf. Bovine Proc. 1986;18:109–12.
44. Cole NA, Camp TH, Rowe LD Jr, Stevens DG, Hutcheson DP. Effect of transport on feeder calves. Am J Vet Res. 1988;49(2):178–83. PMID: 3348528.
45. Crookshank HR, Elissalde MH, White RG, Clanton DC, Smalley HE. Effect of transportation and handling of calves upon blood serum composition. J Anim Sci. 1979;48(3):430–5. https://doi.org/10.2527/jas1979.483430x. PMID: 528410.
46. Cummins JM, Rosenquist BD. Effect of hydrocortisone on the interferon response of calves infected with infectious bovine rhinotracheitis virus. Am J Vet Res. 1977;38(8):1163–6.
47. Purdy CW, Richards AB, Foster GS. Market stress-associated changes in serum complement activity in feeder calves. Am J Vet Res. 1991;52(11):1842–7. PMID: 1785726.
48. Damtew A, Erega Y, Ebrahim H, Tsegaye S, Msigie D. The effect of long distance transportation stress on cattle: a review. Biomed. J Sci Tech Res. 2018;09008:1–5.
49. Chen Y, Arsenault R, Napper S, Griebel P. Models and methods to investigate acute stress responses in cattle. Animals(Basel). 2015;5(4):1268–95.
50. Heiser A, McCarthy A, Wedlock N, et al. Grazing dairy cows had decreased interferon-γ, tumor necrosis factor, and interleukin-17, and increased expression of interleukin-10 during the first week after calving. J Dairy Sci. 2015;98(2):937–46.
51. Nagahata H, Ogawa A, Sanada Y, Noda H, Yamamoto S. Peripartum changes in antibody producing capability of lymphocytes from dairy cows. Vet Q. 1992;14(1):39–40.
52. Kehrli ME Jr, Nonnecke BJ, Roth JA. Alterations in bovine lymphocyte function during the periparturient period. Am J Vet Res. 1989;50(2):215–20.
53. Van Kampen C, Mallard BA. Effects of peripartum stress and health on circulating bovine lymphocyte subsets. Vet Immunol Immunopathol. 1997;59(1–2):79–91.
54. Ishikawa H, Shirahata T, Hasegawa K. Interferon-gamma production of mitogen stimulated peripheral lymphocytes in perinatal cows. J Vet Med Sci. 1994;56(4):735–8.
55. Walz PH, Montgomery T, Passler T, Riddell KP, Braden TD, Zhang Y, Galik PK, Zuidhof S. Comparison of reproductive performance of primiparous dairy cattle following revaccination with either modified-live or killed multivalent viral vaccines in early lactation. J Dairy Sci. 2015;98(12):8753–63. https://doi.org/10.3168/jds.2015-9760. Epub 2015 Oct 9. PMID: 26454300.
56. Cortese VS, Woolums A, Thoresen M, Pinedo PJ, Short T. Mucosal immune responses in peri-parturient dairy cattle. Vet Microbio. 2024;298:110201., ISSN 0378-1135. https://doi.org/10.1016/j.vetmic.2024.110201.
57. Cortese VS, Woolums A, Hurley DJ, Berghaus R, Bernard JK, Short TH. Comparison of interferon and bovine herpesvirus-1-specific IgA levels in nasal secretions of dairy cattle

administered an intranasal modified live viral vaccine prior to calving or on the day of calving. Vet Immunol Immunopath. 2017;187:35–41.
58. Cortese VS, Woolums A, Karisch BB, Short TH, Thoresen M, Badial P. Systemic and local immune responses of beef calves vaccinated post-transportation and at the time of a mild respiratory tract infection. Bov Pract. 2020;54(1):58–65.
59. Cortese VS, Pinedo PJ, Manriquez D, Velasquez-Munoz A, Solano G, Short TH, Cleale R, Edwards G, Montgomery T, Pedraza JR, Bachtell R. Effect of periparturient intranasal vaccination on post parturient health parameters in holstein cows. CDVS. 2020;3(4):318–28. https://doi.org/10.32474/CDVS.2020.03.000167.
60. Step DL, Krehbiel CR, Hixon C, Blanding MR, Hilbig DR, Cortese VS, Short TS. Evaluation of commercially available multivalent modified-live viral vaccines on health and performance in feedlot cattle. J Vaccines Vaccination. 2015;1(3):1–10.
61. Albas A, Fontolan OL, Pardo PE, Bremer NH, Sartori A. Interval between first dose and booster affected antibody production in cattle vaccinated against rabies. J Venomous Anim Toxins Includ Trop Dis. 2006;12:476–86.
62. Cortese VS, Gallo GF, Cleary DL, Galvin JE, Leyh RD. Efficacy of a flexible schedule for administration of a Leptospira borgpetersenii serovar Hardjo bacterin to beef calves. Am J Vet Res. 2014;75(5):507–12.
63. Cortese VS, Seeger JT, Trejo C, Short TH. Impact of maternal antibody and concurrent vaccination on serologic responses to clostridial vaccination in calves. Arch Microbiol Immunol. 2019;3(4):151–60.
64. Mueller D, Noxon JO. Anaphylaxis: pathophysiology and treatment. Compend Contin Educ Pract Vet. 1990;12(2):157–70.
65. Rude TA. Postvaccination Type I Hypersensitivity in Cattle. Agri-Practice. 1990;11(3):29–34.
66. Johansen KA, Wannameuhler M, Rosenbusch RF. Biological reactivity of *Moraxella bovis* lipopolysaccharide. Am J Vet Res. 1990;51(1):46–51.
67. Schuster DE, Harmon RJ, Jackson JA, Hemken RW. Reduced lactational performance following intravenous endotoxin administration to dairy cows. J Dairy Sci. 1991;74:3407–11.
68. Henderson B, Wilson M. Modulins: a new class of cytokine-inducing, pro-inflamatory bacterial virulence factor. Inflamm Res. 1995;44:187–97.
69. Rietschel ET, Brade H. Bacterial endotoxins. Sci Am. 1992;267:55–61.
70. Richeson JT, Hughes HD, Broadway PR, Carroll JA. Vaccination management of beef cattle: delayed vaccination and endotoxin stacking. Vet Clin North Am Food Anim Pract. 2019;35(3):575–92. https://doi.org/10.1016/j.cvfa.2019.07.003. PMID: 31590903; PMCID: PMC7125876.
71. Roth JA. Mechanistic bases for adverse vaccine reactions and vaccine failures. Adv Vet Med. 1999;41:681–700. https://doi.org/10.1016/s0065-3519(99)80053-6. PMID: 9890054; PMCID: PMC7149317.
72. Cussler K, Godau H, Gyra H. Investigation of the endotoxin content of veterinary vaccines. Untersuchungen zum Endotoxingehalt von Tierimpfstoffen. ALTEX. 1994;11(5):24–9.
73. Belhadj Slimen I, Najar T, Ghram A, Abdrrabba M. Heat stress effects on livestock: molecular, cellular and metabolic aspects, a review. J Anim Physiol Anim Nutr. 2016;100:401–12. https://doi.org/10.1111/jpn.12379.
74. Reisinger N, Emsenhuber C, Doupovec B, Mayer E, Schatzmayr G, Nagl V, Grenier B. Endotoxin translocation and gut inflammation are increased in broiler chickens receiving an oral lipopolysaccharide (LPS) bolus during heat stress. Toxins. 2020;12(10):622. https://doi.org/10.3390/toxins12100622.
75. Cheng H, Freire R, Pajor EA. Endotoxin stress responses in chickens from different genetic lines. 1. Sickness, behavioral, and physical responses. Poultry science. 2004;83:707–15. https://doi.org/10.1093/ps/83.5.707.
76. Smit LAM, Heederik D, Doekes G, Krop EJM, Rijkers GT, Wouters IM. Ex vivo cytokine release reflects sensitivity to occupational endotoxin exposure. Eur Respir J. 2009;34(4):795–802. https://doi.org/10.1183/09031936.00161908.

77. Falcon RMG, Caoili SEC. Immunologic, genetic, and ecological interplay of factors involved in allergic diseases. Front Allergy. 2023;4:1215616. https://doi.org/10.3389/falgy.2023.1215616. PMID: 37601647; PMCID: PMC10435091.
78. Bamouh Z, Hamdi J, Fellahi S, Khayi S, Jazouli M, Tadlaoui KO, Fihri OF, Tuppurainen E, Elharrak M. Investigation of post vaccination reactions of two live attenuated vaccines against lumpy skin disease of cattle. Vaccines (Basel). 2021;9(6):621. https://doi.org/10.3390/vaccines9060621. PMID: 34201339; PMCID: PMC8226854.
79. Garcia-Pintos C, Riet-Correa F, Menchaca A. Effect of foot-and-mouth disease vaccine on pregnancy failure in beef cows. Front Vet Sci. 2021;8:761304. https://doi.org/10.3389/fvets.2021.761304. PMID: 34869734; PMCID: PMC8633299.
80. O'Toole D, Steadman L, Raisbeck M, Torpy R. Myositis, lameness, and recumbency after use of water-in-oil adjuvanted vaccines in near-term beef cattle. J Vet Diagn Invest. 2005;17:23–31.
81. Cresswell E, Remnant J, Butterworth A, Wapenaar W. Injection-site lesion prevalence and potential risk factors in UK beef cattle. Vet Rec. 2017;180(3):70. https://doi.org/10.1136/vr.103778.
82. Woodland DL. Jump-starting the immune system: prime-boosting comes of age. Trends Immunol. 2004;25(2):98–104. https://doi.org/10.1016/j.it.2003.11.009.
83. Kardani K, Bolhassani A, Shahbazi S. Prime-boost vaccine strategy against viral infections: Mechanisms and benefits. Vaccine. 2016;34(4):413–23. https://doi.org/10.1016/j.vaccine.2015.11.062. Epub 2015 Dec 13. PMID: 2669156.
84. Ramshaw IA, Ramsay AJ. The prime-boost strategy: exciting prospects for improved vaccination. Immunol Today. 2000;21:163–5.
85. Cortese VS, Seeger JT, Trejo C, Short TH. Antibody responses to BHV-1 vaccination in neonatal calves and in prime-boost programs EC veterinary. Science. 2020;5(3):1–11.
86. Ellis J, Gow S, Berenik A, Lacoste S, Erickson N. Comparative efficacy of modified-live and inactivated vaccines in boosting responses to bovine respiratory syncytial virus following neonatal mucosal priming of beef calves. Can Vet J. 2018;59(12):1311–9. PMID: 30532289; PMCID: PMC6237255.
87. Erickson N, Godson D, Gow S, Lacoste S, Waldner C, Ellis J. Comparative efficacy of modified-live and inactivated vaccines in boosting disease-sparing responses to bovine viral diarrhea virus challenge in neonatally mucosally primed weanling beef calves. Can Vet J. 2023;64(4):321–8. PMID: 37008637; PMCID: PMC10031784.
88. Erickson NEN, April S, Campbell JR, Homerosky E, Ware T, Dorin C, Waldner CL, Ellis JA. Comparison of postweaning bovine respiratory disease treatment rates between non-vaccinated control beef calves and calves variably primed and boosted using commercially available bovine coronavirus vaccines. Can Vet J. 2024;65(6):581–6. PMID: 38827595; PMCID: PMC11132172.
89. Erickson N, Waldner C, Snyder E, Bravo Araya M, Sniatynski M, Ellis J. Comparative efficacy of modified-live and inactivated vaccines in boosting responses to bovine respiratory syncytial virus, bovine parainfluenza virus Type 3, and bovine coronavirus following neonatal mucosal priming of beef calves. Can Vet J. 2024;65(8):791–801. PMID: 39091482; PMCID: PMC11265827.
90. Palgen JL, Feraoun Y, Dzangué-Tchoupou G, Joly C, Martinon F, Le Grand R, Beignon AS. Optimize prime/boost vaccine strategies: trained immunity as a new player in the game. Front Immunol. 2021;12:612747. https://doi.org/10.3389/fimmu.2021.612747. PMID: 33763063; PMCID: PMC7982481.
91. de Oliveira Santos FA, Lincopan N, De Gaspari E. Evaluation of intranasal and subcutaneous route of immunization in neonatal mice using DODAB-BF as adjuvant with outer membrane vesicles of Neisseria meningitis B. Immunobiology. 2018;223(12):750–60. https://doi.org/10.1016/j.imbio.2018.07.021. Epub 2018 Jul 19. PMID: 30055864.
92. Fiorino F, Pettini E, Pozzi G, Medaglini D, Ciabattini A. Prime-boost strategies in mucosal immunization affect local IgA production and the type of th response. Front Immunol.

2013;4:128. https://doi.org/10.3389/fimmu.2013.00128. PMID: 23755051; PMCID: PMC3665932.

93. Eo SK, Gierynska M, Kamar AA, Rouse BT. Prime-boost immunization with DNA vaccine: mucosal route of administration changes the rules. J Immunol. 2001;166(9):5473–9. https://doi.org/10.4049/jimmunol.166.9.5473.
94. Erickson NEN, Berenik A, Lardner H, Lacoste S, Campbell J, Gow S, Waldner C, Ellis J. Evaluation of bovine respiratory syncytial virus (BRSV) and bovine herpesvirus (BHV) specific antibody responses between heterologous and homologous prime-boost vaccinated western Canadian beef calves. Can Vet J. 2021;62(1):37–44. PMID: 33390597; PMCID: PMC7739395.
95. Sapkota B, Saud B, Shrestha R, Al-Fahad D, Sah R, Shrestha S, Rodriguez-Morales AJ. Heterologous prime-boost strategies for COVID-19 vaccines. J Travel Med. 2022;29(3):taab191. https://doi.org/10.1093/jtm/taab191. PMID: 34918097; PMCID: PMC8754745.
96. Bernelin-Cottet C, Urien C, Stubsrud E, Jakob V, Bouguyon E, Bordet E, Barc C, Boulesteix O, Contreras V, Barnier-Quer C, Collin N, Trus I, Nauwynck H, Bertho N, Schwartz-Cornil I. A DNA-modified live vaccine prime-boost strategy broadens the T-cell response and enhances the antibody response against the porcine reproductive and respiratory syndrome virus. Viruses. 2019;11(6):551. https://doi.org/10.3390/v11060551. PMID: 31207934; PMCID: PMC6630347.
97. Walz PH, Givens MD, Rodning SP, Riddell KP. Evaluation of reproductive protection against bovine viral diarrhea virus and bovine herpesvirus-1 afforded by annual revaccination with modified-live viral or combination modified-live/killed viral vaccines after primary vaccination with modified-live viral vaccine. Vaccine. 2017;35(7):1046–54. https://doi.org/10.1016/j.vaccine.2017.01.006.
98. Khalifa M, El-Deeb A, Zeidan S, Hussein H, Abu-El-Naga H. Enhanced protection against FMDV in cattle after prime- boost vaccination based on mucosal and inactivated FMD vaccine. Vet Microbio. 2017;210:1–7. https://doi.org/10.1016/j.vetmic.2017.08.014.
99. Alborali GL, Ruggeri J, Pesciaroli M, et al. Prime-boost vaccination with attenuated Salmonella Typhimurium ΔznuABC and inactivated Salmonella choleraesuis is protective against Salmonella choleraesuis challenge infection in piglets. BMC Vet Res. 2017;13(1):284. Published 2017 Sep 11. https://doi.org/10.1186/s12917-017-1202-5.
100. Asadi Karam MR, Shirzad AM, Habibi M, Bouzari S. A heterologous prime-boost route of vaccination based on the truncated MrpH adhesin and adjuvant properties of the flagellin from Proteus mirabilis against urinary tract infections. Int Immunopharmacol. 2018;58:40–7. https://doi.org/10.1016/j.intimp.2018.03.009.
101. Van Reeth K, Mancera Gracia JC, Trus I, Sys L, Claes G, Versnaeyen V, Cox E, Krammer F, Qiu Y. Heterologous prime-boost vaccination with H3N2 influenza viruses of swine favors cross-clade antibody responses and protection. NPJ Vaccines. 2017;2(11):10.1038/s41541-017-0012-x.
102. Mapletoft JW, Latimer L, Babiuk LA, van Drunen Littel-van den Hurk S. Intranasal immunization of mice with a bovine respiratory syncytial virus vaccine induces superior immunity and protection compared to those by subcutaneous delivery or combinations of intranasal and subcutaneous prime-boost strategies. Clin Vaccine Immunol. 2010;17(1):23–35. https://doi.org/10.1128/CVI.00250-09. Epub 2009 Oct 28. PMID: 19864487; PMCID: PMC2812083.
103. Phuensan P, Sirimongkolkasem J, Tantawichien T, Phannajit J, Kerr SJ, Hansasuta P, Chantharit P, Wongsa A, Fuengfoo P, Chittinandana A, Vareesangthip K, Chayakulkeeree M, Jangsirikul S, Schmidt A, Wanvimonsuk K, Winichakoon P, Kajeekul R, Prayoonwiwat W, Rerknimitr R. Immunogenicity and safety of heterologous versus homologous prime-boost schedules with inactivated and adenoviral vectored SARS-CoV-2 vaccines - A prospective multi-center study. Heliyon. 2023;10(1):e23246. https://doi.org/10.1016/j.heliyon.2023.e23246. PMID: 38163241; PMCID: PMC10756999.

104. Frelinger JA. Introduction. In: Frelinger JA, editor. Immunodominance: the choice of the immune system. 1st ed. Wiley-VCH Verlag GmbH; 2005.; ISBN:9783527608027. https://doi.org/10.1002/3527608028.
105. Akram A, Inman RD. Immunodominance: a pivotal principle in host response to viral infections. Clin Immunol. 2012;143(2):99–115. https://doi.org/10.1016/j.clim.2012.01.015.
106. Angeletti D, Gibbs J, Angel M, Kosik I, Hickman HD, Frank GM, Das SR, Wheatley AK, Prabhakaran M, Leggat DJ, McDermott AB, Yewdell JW. Defining B cell immunodominance to viruses. Nat Immunol. 2017;18:456–63. https://doi.org/10.1038/ni.3680.
107. Caradonna TM, Schmidt AG. Protein engineering strategies for rational immunogen design. NPJ Vaccines. 2021;691540. https://doi.org/10.1038/s41541-021-00417-1.
108. Kim PS, Lee PP, Levy D. A theory of immunodominance and adaptive regulation. Bull Math Biol. 2011;73(7):1645–65. https://doi.org/10.1007/s11538-010-9585-5. Epub 2010 Oct 1. PMID: 20886303; PMCID: PMC3865720.
109. Kim PS, Lee PP, Levy D. Basic principles in modeling adaptive regulation and immunodominance. In: Ledzewicz U, Schättler H, Friedman A, Kashdan E, editors. Mathematical methods and models in biomedicine. Lecture notes on mathematical modelling in the life sciences. New York: Springer; 2013. https://doi.org/10.1007/978-1-4614-4178-6_2.
110. Lindahl G. Subdominance in antibody responses: implications for vaccine development. Microbiol Mol Biol Rev. 2020;85(1):e00078–20. https://doi.org/10.1128/MMBR.00078-20. PMID: 33239435; PMCID: PMC7709521.
111. Harland RJ, Potter AA, van Drunen-Littel-van den Hurk S, Van Donkersgoed J, Parker MD, Zamb TJ, Janzen ED. The effect of subunit or modified live bovine herpesvirus-1 vaccines on the efficacy of a recombinant Pasteurella haemolytica vaccine for the prevention of respiratory disease in feedlot calves. Can Vet J. 1992;33(11):734–41. PMID: 17424116; PMCID: PMC1481421.
112. Cortese VS, Seeger JT, Stokka GL, Hunsaker BD, Lardy GP, Weigel DJ, Brumbaugh GW. Serologic response to Mannheimia haemolytica in calves concurrently inoculated with inactivated or modified-live preparations of M. haemolytica and viral combination vaccines containing modified-live bovine herpesvirus type 1. Am J Vet Res. 2011;72(11):1541–9.
113. Cortese VS, Hankins K, Holland R, Syvrud K. Serologic responses of West Nile Virus seronegative mature horses to West Nile Virus vaccines JEVS. 2013;33(12):1101–5.
114. Madapong A, Saeng-chuto K, Tantituvanont A, et al. Using a concurrent challenge with porcine circovirus 2 and porcine reproductive and respiratory syndrome virus to compare swine vaccination programs. Sci Rep. 2022;12:15524. https://doi.org/10.1038/s41598-022-19529-2.
115. Munks MW, Hill AB. Immunodominance in the T-cell response to herpesviruses. In: Frelinger JA, editor. Immunodominance: the choice of the immune system. 1st ed. Wiley-VCH Verlag GmbH; 2005. p. 255–83. ISBN:9783527608027. https://doi.org/10.1002/3527608028.
116. American Association of Bovine Practitioners, AABP (2021). http://www.aabp.org/committees/resources/VaccGuidelines2021.pdf.

Appendix 1: Answers to "Your Case" Questions

Chapter 1

1. *How would you have likely determined that the calves had acute versus persistent BVDV infections?*

   Determine those animals that tested positive on a first quantitative polymerase chain reaction (qPCR) for BVDV and negative on the second test, 2 weeks later (transiently infected), compared to those positive on both tests (persistently infected).
2. *What should you discuss with the owner concerning responses to vaccination in this group of calves?*

   Inform the owner that the responses to vaccination may be less than optimal due to the effects of BVDV virus infection in the primary lymphoid organs, ileal Peyer's patches, and thymus

Chapter 2

1. *Based on the clinical history and your necropsy findings, is this owner most likely to be correct in his "internet diagnosis" of anaphylaxis? Why or why not?*

   This is unlikely to be a case of anaphylaxis. Although the lungs are the target for anaphylactic reactions in cattle, this type of allergic (type 1 hypersensitivity) reaction would generally occur within minutes, and not many hours, after exposure. Moreover, these genetically restricted reactions are almost never going to affect an entire group of animals, but rather are rare.
2. *What is the most likely immunological mechanism involved in this case?*

   Given the history, extent and nature of the clinical signs, and postmortem findings, this case is most likely to be an example of the effects of a cytokine storm or "cytokine intoxication" that resulted from a high concentration of PAMPs, perhaps endotoxin from *H. somni* or other vaccine components.

J. Ellis, V. Cortese, *Practical Bovine Immunology*,
https://doi.org/10.1007/978-3-032-15031-8

Chapter 3

1. *What do low CT values on a diagnostic PCR test report indicate? Why?*

   Lower CT or "cycle threshold" values indicate more virus in the sample (the more virus genetic material in the sample, the fewer cycles needed to detect).
2. *From the perspective of protective antibody responses alone, why do you think that the vaccine that stimulated the lower concentration of BRSV-specific antibody apparently provided better clinical protection?*

   The antibody that is produced in response to the conventional modified-live vaccine probably has more neutralizing capability, at least in part due to preservation of conformational determinants on the viral envelope glycoproteins of the virus. The adjuvanted protein subunit vaccine could be stimulating the production of higher amounts of antibody to epitopes that are not involved in neutralization of the virus.
3. *What does the type of test that is used to quantitate virus-specific antibody tell you about the functionality of the antibody that is being measured?*

   Bioassays such as neutralization tests or fusion inhibition tests usually use intact viruses and measure functional responses against envelope glycoproteins; the ability of antibodies to block these functions. ELISA tests using whole virus adsorb the virus to plastic plates, dry the virus onto the plate, and often use a fixative, such as acetone. This process can destroy conformational determinants and expose internal virus proteins that are not involved in neutralization. So, an ELISA test can measure antibodies to epitopes that are not important as targets for protective antibody responses. The results of bioassays and ELISA tests are not necessarily directly correlated.

Chapter 4

1. *You're thinking about the type of vaccine needed to be effective against B. abortus. Since Brucella spp. are bacteria, should not an antibody response be sufficient? Why do we need a modified-live vaccine to begin with?*

   Brucella spp. are facultative intracellular pathogens. Antibodies can aid in the "neutralization" or elimination of extracellular bacteria; however, similarly to the situation with *Mycobacteria* spp., it is thought that cell-mediated immune (CMI) responses are required to control *Brucella* spp. Conventionally, CMI responses are associated with modified-live vaccines, but it is not that simple, as discussed in answers 2 and 3.
2. *What specific types of immune responses would you expect to get in response to the RB-15 vaccine? Would it be the same or different with a subunit vaccine? Can an inactivated or subunit vaccine stimulate a cell-mediated or "CMI" response? Why or why not?*

   Generally speaking, MLV vaccines stimulate a broader immune response than inactivated or subunit vaccines. B cells can recognize epitopes on the surface of RB-15 bacteria or subunit proteins. As well, when the bacteria in RB-15 or the proteins in the subunit vaccine are phagocytized or engulfed by antigen-presenting cells such as dendritic cells, they are processed, and the resulting peptides are presented to CD4+ T cells in association with MHC-II molecules. Cytokines from these helper T cells can help in the maturation of B cells and in the production of antibodies. These stimulated cells can also secrete Th1-like cytokines, importantly INF-γ, that can activate macrophages to more effectively kill intracellular bacteria. This is one type of a "CMI" reaction. However, "dead" proteins (not in their native conformation and not processed via the endogenous pathway by antigen-presenting cells), whether whole bacteria or subunits, together with conventional adjuvants, such as oil-based adjuvants, CANNOT, stimulate CD8+ cytotoxic T cells, which need to see their specific antigen in association with MHC-I molecules. This requires the "infection" of cells in the animal and processing of antigens through the endogenous pathway of antigen presentation, ultimately involving the MHC-I molecules.

3. *Could a skin fold test be used to monitor response to B. abortus vaccine? Why or why not? Answering the wildlife biologist's question, what specific types of immune responses are occurring in the lump in a positive skin fold test? Would a test for antibody be just as good?*

   A skin fold test or assessment of delayed-type hypersensitivity could be used to measure CMI responses with the appropriate Brucella antigen preparation, similar to purified protein derivative from *Mycobacteria* spp. The primary cells in a DTH reaction are CD4+ T cells that secrete Th-1-like cytokines, notably IFN-γ, and macrophages that have been activated by IFN-γ. CD8+ T cells and natural killer cells play a minor role. Traditionally, antibody tests (detailed in the next chapter) have been used to diagnose *Brucella* spp. infections or exposure. Thus, this test could be used to assess the immune response to vaccines. Measurement of interferon gamma release from T cells from infected animals (detailed in the next chapter) has also been used to diagnose *M. bovis* infections and could be used for *Brucella* spp. as well.

Chapter 5

1. *Would an apparent twofold difference in response to the two vaccines be indicative of a significant difference in responses to the two vaccines?*

   No, a doubling dilution would not generally be considered evidence of seroconversion or a significant difference. In your case, the calves that received the "old" vaccine apparently seroconverted; the calves that received the "new" vaccine did not. But as can happen, there does not appear to be a difference between the two groups after vaccination.

2. *If you decide, for financial purposes, to change diagnostic laboratories, should you compare the VN results from two different laboratories, assuming that they use the same standard procedures? Why or why not? What about assays conducted on two different days in the same laboratory?*

No, because of, often unintended, biological variation in the way VN tests are performed, you should not compare VN results among laboratories. And, from a practical standpoint, there can be intra-lab variation (e.g., on different days); you should submit acute and convalescent samples simultaneously so that they can be directly compared in the same set of assays.

3. *Some diagnostic laboratories use virus neutralization tests to quantitate virus-specific antibody responses, and others use ELISA tests. What is the difference in the way the tests are done and the way the results are determined and reported?*

   Virus neutralization tests are generally done using serial dilutions of serum, and results are reported as a "titer," the last dilution of serum that prevents viral plaque formation (CPE). This test measures the ability of antibodies in the sample to "neutralize" the virus, usually by blocking infection. It is, by definition, a measure of a functional response. In contrast, an ELISA is usually performed on one standard dilution, and results are reported as units of activity, or simply, positive or negative. ELISAs indicate the binding of an antibody to an epitope(s) on the virus. Binding to this epitope may or may not result in neutralization of the virus.

Chapter 6

1. *Based on history and necropsy, what is your presumptive diagnosis?*

   The necropsy does not support the owner's diagnosis of pneumonia. The tracheal, nasal, and laryngeal lesions are consistent with acute respiratory BHV-1 infection. However, the severity of the disease is not consistent with a BHV-1 infection (see Chap. 6, reference 81). The ulcers in one of the calves suggest a co-infection with BHV-1 and BVDV.

2. *Based on your diagnosis, how do you proceed?*

   The remaining animals are vaccinated with an intranasal MLV three-way viral vaccine (BHV-1, PI3, and BRSV) and an injectable MLV BVDV vaccine. A metaphylactic dose of tulathromycin is also given. While administration of vaccine in the face of an outbreak is somewhat controversial, it is routinely done by many (particularly the intranasal) and in this situation is your potential way to slow down the BVDV spread and decrease the BHV-1 severity. The rapid release of interferon after intranasal BHV-1 vaccination has been well published.

3. *How do you explain the rapid and high mortality rate in the infected cattle?*

   PCR results are positive for both BHV-1 and BVD. A total of 54 of the 100 purchased cattle became ill. Twenty of these calves died or were euthanized, giving a final mortality rate of 37%. None of the home-raised cattle got sick, and within 7 days of vaccination, no further sick cattle were seen. A skin sample (ear notch) for BVDV immunohistochemistry was performed, but no BVDV persistently infected cattle were identified. It was assumed that the PI calf may have been among the 20 calves that had perished. You explain to the owner that the immune suppression due to the BVDV infection dramatically increased the severity of the BHV-1 infection (see Chap. 6, reference 82). You also inform him that not waiting to vaccinate the cattle may have decreased the losses.

Chapter 7

1. *How do you start to diagnose the underlying cause of the scours outbreak?*
   Laboratory results from calves brought into the clinic for treatment Serum total proteins 7.5–8.0 g/dl. Cryptosporidia, Rotavirus, and coronavirus positive on fecal samples. As a follow-up question, why might these results be misleading? Since calves being brought to the clinic are dehydrated, the total proteins are not accurate.
2. *What follow-up testing do you do based on the initial results?*
   Random serum total proteins on 2–7-day-old calves range from 4.8 to 5.6 g/dL; 28% are below 5.1 g/dL. Blood samples showed low vitamin E and marginal selenium levels in three out of five cows and five out of five heifers. The rancher noticed that calves were often slow to stand and nurse. No heat abatement was seen in the pastures.
3. *What are your recommendations to control this outbreak and prevent it next year?*
   Since the primary problem is the failure of passive transfer. It may be too late to impact the quality this year; however, a vitamin E/selenium injection to the cows and newborn calves may have some benefit. Pasture rotation to decrease pathogen exposure is important for this year and for future years, as well as correcting the trace mineral deficiency, since the low vitamin E and selenium were contributing to both the poorer quality of the colostrum and the delayed time to nurse in the calves. Adding some form of heat abatement for the cattle on pasture may also help improve colostral quality.

Chapter 8

1. *Which result is misleading?*
   Since the calves are getting an oral MLV rotavirus/coronavirus vaccine at the dairy before going to the calf ranch, the coronavirus positive result may be from the vaccine. However, the myriads of digestive and respiratory pathogens identified lean toward immune system dysfunction.
2. *What is the primary problem?*
   Calves are fed a milk-based milk replacer with 20% crude protein and 12% fat (13% total solids), at a rate of two quarts twice a day. You determine that the primary problem is energy deficiency with a secondary immune system shutdown. Cold stress exacerbates energy deficiency. The economy milk replacer fat content is too low, and the protein content is marginal, particularly in cold weather.

3. *What would you look for to confirm your diagnosis?*

   While necropsy results are typical for diarrhea (greenish fluid-filled large intestines) and pneumonia (fibrinonecrotic pneumonia with extensive consolidation and discoloration of cranioventral lungs with fibrinous pleuritis), it is the absence of fat present around the heart and kidneys on all calves that confirms your diagnosis.

Chapter 9

1. *What is your presumptive diagnosis?*

   Your tentative diagnosis is heavy parasitism. Your physical examination does not tell what parasite it is.
2. *What diagnostic tests do you perform?*

   CBC and differential indicate anemia and hypoproteinemia in the most severely affected heifers. There are also increases in both eosinophils and neutrophils in the blood. Fecal flotation results from several samples include a few coccidia eggs and numerous trichostrongyle eggs. The eggs were determined to be Haemonchus.
3. *What is your treatment plan?*

   You would like to use a long-acting Avermectin dewormer; however, this is not permitted in organic beef operations. Since the animals are replacement heifers and disease has been documented, approval is obtained to use fenbendazole oral paste. After treatment, all heifers are moved to an ungrazed pasture. Three weaker heifers are also given a transfusion. Cattle are provided a grain supplement daily for 30 days to assist in regaining lost weight. Pasture management is discussed for future consideration.

Chapter 10

Questions

1. *Where do you start to work up this complex problem?*

   Due to the severity of the reproductive issues, the owner agrees to a complete diagnostic workup. You collect whole blood, serum, and liver biopsies from five cows with infertility issues. Ten cows with infertility issues and 10 bred cows have paired serum samples and are tested for BVD, BHV-1 (VN titers), and Leptospira (MAT). Vaginal scoping of infertility cases showed that no lesions or abnormal discharges were observed. Vaginal cultures from embryonic loss cases were collected. Silage was tested for mycotoxins.

   Results include *Histophilus somni* cultured from one cow, mycotoxins in silage were within acceptable ranges, selenium whole blood levels averaged 210 μg/L, none below 180 μg/L, liver copper levels averaged 304 mg/kg, none below 200 mg/kg, and zinc serum levels averaged 1.0 mg/L (all considered within normal ranges). No differences were seen in titers between the two groups. BVDV titers ranged from 1:256 to 1:2048, BHV-1 1:64 to 1:512. Leptospira titers ranged from 0 to 1000. You consider these to be normal vaccination titers.

2. *Based on initial diagnostics, what do you recommend?*

   Since there is nothing obvious from the diagnostic testing, you focus on breeding management. Changes include:

   (a) Switching to a double ovsynch program
   (b) Double sheathing all inseminations
   (c) Instituting a *H. somni* vaccination program

3. *What results do you anticipate within 6 months on the program?*

   You expect to see an improvement in reproductive indices, particularly first service conception rates, decreasing EED rates, and culls due to reproductive failure. However, no improvement is seen, and the herd did not have enough replacement heifers due to the abnormally high cull rate and had to purchase additional bred heifers.

4. *If unsatisfactory results after 6 months, what further diagnostics would you run?*

   A follow-up diagnostic plan is formulated. In the case of negative BVD serology, bulk tank BVDV PCRs are scheduled quarterly for the next year. A clean-up bull is used for problem breeders for 3 months to compare results. A Leptospira testing procedure was done. Twenty cows (10 infertility and 10 EED) were administered furosemide, and urine samples were collected for Leptospira PCR and culture.

   Results include two negative BVDV bulk tank samples to date and minimal improvement in breeding results from the cleanup bull. Out of 20, 16 cows were identified as having *Leptospira borgpetersenii* Hardjo-bovis bacteria in their urine.

5. *Based on further testing, what changes would you make to the program?*

   With a diagnosis of Leptospira reproductive infections, changes include:

   (a) Instituting a Leptospira borgpetersenii Hardjo-bovis vaccination program with a vaccine that has reproductive labels
   (b) Oxytetracycline administration to each cow at the cessation of milk
   (c) Removal of the cleanup bull
   (d) No further bulk tank BVDV OCR testing

Final Outcome

After 6 months on this program, there is a slight improvement in reproductive numbers. Follow-up testing still showed 10 out of 20 cows had *Leptospira borgpetersenii* Hardjo-bovis bacteria in their urine. Due to articles showing *Leptospira borgpetersenii* Hardjo-bovis is cleared from urinary and reproductive tracts by cephalosporins [101], the owner opted to treat the entire herd with a dose of cephalosporins. Reproduction returned to normal in the herd after the antibiotic treatment. The herd remained negative for Leptospira in the urine on follow-up testing 3 months and 12 months after the treatment and remained on the vaccination program.

Chapter 11

1. *What is your tentative diagnosis? How do you confirm it?*
   Although you have not seen cases before, your diagnosis is acute endotoxic coliform mastitis. Since the herd is pasture-based, it is most likely due to *E. coli*. This is confirmed by cultures of milk samples from affected quarters.
2. *How do you treat the recumbent cows? What do you anticipate for an outcome?*
   You treat the cows with intravenous fluids, including calcium, antihistamines, corticosteroids, and antibiotics. Two of the cows can rise after treatment, but one remains recumbent. You instruct the manager to have the infected quarters milked every 2 h. While you anticipate that the two cows will survive the episode, severe damage to their quarters makes the future production from those quarters questionable. The outcome of the cow's unable to rise is unknown.
3. *Why is the dairy experiencing this problem?*
   Unknown to you, the dairy discontinued the use of a core endotoxin vaccination program. The rationale was that they had *E. coli* vaccine in their scours vaccination program. The dairy does not use a teat sealant after milking.
4. *The following day, the dairy finds two more cows with hard quarters, elevated temperatures, and anorexia. What is your course of action to prevent new cases?*
   The core endotoxin vaccine is put back into the program, and a teat sealant is recommended to be used during times when the pastures may become muddy. Pasture management and pre-milking procedures are revisited.

Chapter 12

1. *What does a BRIX value indicate, and how is it measured?*
   A Brix refractometer measures the Brix value, which represents the percentage of total soluble solids in a liquid solution. In the context of colostrum quality in cattle, this primarily reflects the concentration of immunoglobulins (primarily IgG1), along with other solids such as proteins, sugars, and minerals. While originally developed for measuring sugar content in fruit juices and wine, the Brix scale has proven useful in veterinary applications because higher Brix readings in colostrum generally correlate with higher IgG levels. A Brix reading of 22% or higher is typically considered indicative of high-quality colostrum suitable for newborn calves. In contrast, IgG is measured specifically using radial immunodiffusion (RID).
2. *How is total serum protein in calves determined? How does it relate to IgG concentrations? What is considered evidence of adequate passive transfer?*
   Total serum protein (TSP) in calves is commonly measured 24–48 h after birth using a refractometer to assess the success of passive transfer. TSP reflects the concentration of proteins in the blood, including immunoglobulin G (IgG1), which is the key antibody absorbed from colostrum. Although TSP is an indirect measure, it correlates well with IgG levels. A TSP level of $\geq$5.5 g/dL and an IgG concentration of $\geq$10 g/L (measured by RID) are considered indicators of successful passive transfer.

3. *Why are calves with bacterial pneumonia "sick," and what is the role of the innate immune system in "sickness behavior"?*

   Calves with bacterial pneumonia become "sick" largely because of the innate response. It responds rapidly by recognizing common viral and bacterial components (PAMPs), unique to microbes and often called "danger signals," through pattern recognition receptors (PRRs, e.g., Toll-like receptors) on innate immune cells such as macrophages and neutrophils. These cells release pro-inflammatory cytokines (e.g., IL-1 and TNF-α) that cause fever, loss of appetite, and lethargy—classic signs of illness. Neutrophils also migrate into the lungs to engulf and kill bacteria, but in doing so, they release enzymes and reactive oxygen species that can damage lung tissue, leading to coughing, labored breathing, and reduced oxygen exchange. This immune-driven inflammation is essential for clearing infection but also contributes to the calf's clinical signs of illness. Largely, innate immune-mediated "sickness" is a (pathogen) load phenomenon; a little innate immune response early in infection is protective, whereas a lot in uncontrolled infection is essentially the clinical disease.
4. *Why are intranasal vaccines potentially more efficacious than injectable vaccines, especially in young calves?*

   Intranasal vaccines are considerably less likely to be blocked by maternal antibodies because they primarily stimulate a different part of the immune system than injectable vaccines. Intranasal vaccines work by targeting the mucosal immune system—specifically the nasal-associated lymphoid tissue—which is part of the local adaptive immune response in the respiratory tract. In the absence of inflammation, there is only a small amount of maternal IgG1 in the upper respiratory tract, so it is less likely to neutralize vaccine viruses and interfere with a response. As a result, intranasal vaccines can effectively stimulate local IgA production and cellular immunity in the nasal passages, providing early protection against respiratory pathogens even in the presence of circulating maternal antibodies.

Chapter 13

1. *What is your tentative diagnosis?*

   You diagnose a respiratory virus infection with some secondary pneumonia seen in the post-partum cows. Calving stress may be involved.
2. *What do you do next?*

   You obtain deep nasopharyngeal swabs from the three cows with high fever and from one cow with pneumonia. Blood and liver samples are collected for mineral and vitamin analysis. Temperatures are collected on all cows under 30 days in milk twice a week, and any with elevated temperatures are given the cephalosporin. Nasal swabs are PCR negative for any routine viruses. The nasal swab from the cow with pneumonia cultured positive for *Mannheimia hemolytica*. Nutritional panels are normal. Over the next month, the febrile (>104°F) rate is 17%.

3. *Based on the results, what do you recommend?*

   A Mannheimia hemolytica vaccination is added 14 days prior to calving, and a five-way inactivated viral vaccine is added to the vaccination program to be administered at dry off (60 days prior to calving). The cows are currently on an MLV five-way viral vaccine with Leptospira vaccination prior to breeding.
4. *Do you have any further suggestions if the recommendations do not work?*

   During the next 2 months, there is no change in febrile rate or cull rates. Follow-up nasopharyngeal swabs are negative. The inactivated viral vaccine is removed, and an intranasal three-way MLV viral vaccine is administered on the day of calving. Over the course of the next 2 months, only one febrile cow is found. Bi-weekly temperatures are discontinued, and the Mannheimia vaccine is removed. While the cause of the fevers is never discovered, the generic anti-viral stimulation of the nasal immune system by intranasal MLV BHV-1 vaccines is well documented, and you assume that this secondary benefit of the vaccine is controlling an unknown respiratory virus.

Chapter 14

1. *What are your three primary rule-outs for this problem?*

   With the history of thunderstorms and sudden death, lightning cannot be dismissed as a potential cause of death in the heifers. However, a delayed reaction to vaccination or acute toxicity is higher on your list of probabilities.
2. *How can you differentiate between your suspected causes of death and weakness?*

   Necropsies and physical examination should be able to rule out lightning and possibly toxicities. You can find no burn marks on any of the heifers, and the dead heifers are not close together in the pasture. Necropsies on several dead animals show similar lesions. Severe pulmonary edema with copious amounts of mucoid foam in the trachea. No other lesions are seen. While it does not rule out toxicities, the farm workers confirm that nothing has changed in the last 48 hours with feed, treatments, or pasture maintenance. The heifers have been housed in the same area for roughly a month. The necropsies are consistent with an adverse reaction to vaccination. The delayed time following vaccination suggests a delayed hypersensitivity or a gram-negative stacking reaction.
3. *Are there any underlying issues to be explored in the case?*

   You perform trace mineral analysis on three liver samples from necropsied heifers. Selenium levels ranged from 0.7 to 0.9 μg/g (normal range 1.1–5.9 μg/g) and tocopherol levels 8–10 μg/g (normal 7–40 μg/g).
4. *What treatments, if any, can you do for the remaining heifers?*

   Recumbent heifers were treated with flunixin, dexamethasone, and fluids (containing calcium). Eight of the nine treated heifers recovered.

5. *What advice would you give the dairy to avoid the same problem in the future?*
   It was discovered that the heifers were accidentally vaccinated with a modified live five-way viral vaccine and five-way leptospirosis vaccine that also contained a vibrio fraction that added to the Gram-negative vaccine stacking. You redo the vaccination program to remove the Vibrio and Mannheimia vaccines, and vaccination timing is moved to early morning during the summer months (after a discussion on heat stress in cattle). Selenium and vitamin E levels were corrected in the ratio.